FAT

by James Keene

To my wife and family.

Look at my new wife, wading in her black one-piece. Even at seventy-two, she is jaw-dropping: lean, tall and leggy, peach skin delicate without noticeable turkey neck or cottage cheese, and filling out her top with a perked hyperbolic curve as if thirty years younger. Her attractiveness has only intensified as her telomeres have shortened. From a peck-on-cheek childish crush to hormonal teenaged lust to young adult love, her effect was such that it could always erase complicating time and accumulating neuroses. We had finally made it to this beach.

"Bill, honey, come on in, the water is great."

I wave to her. I will join her in a bit, but not before I watch the water lap at her body a bit more. She is the only light on this beach.

There is a topless sunbather a dozen yards to my left who, even in her mid-30's, looks like an overfed cow with two overused udders on her chest that are more Slinky than skin; her breasts were leaking off the flanks making her nipples areola-down in the sand like two embarrassed ostriches. A middle aged

1

man had just walked by me who was either completely naked with his genitals disappeared under belly and thigh rolls, or he had on a too-tight Speedo that had disappeared under belly and thigh rolls. The dozens of swarming kids all had the physiques of aged bowlers and were running to and from the snack bar with cheeks overflowing, as if the rush of hogs around the trough finally filled with the day's slop. My wife in the ocean looks like the size of something everyone else would eat for lunch.

My cell phone starts chiming, and interrupts my ogling. Nearby people glance in my direction. My ring tone is a bleating tuba repeating the same two notes, the soundtrack of Humpty Dumpty ambling down the street, or of any of these other beach-goers trudging through the sand.

"Hello...yes, this is him...hi, Dr. Reebs…okay…he went when?…okay…well, thank you for all of your efforts…we will…okay, goodbye."

There are overweight people populating this country, young and old, but rare is the four hundred pound ninety year old. They just don't last that long. Well, if they do, they're just rotting away in a nursing home unseen, needing constant orderly assistance in turning and feeding, not having felt fresh air or a new person's stare on their skin since their weight was measured in pounds and not in fractions of tons. Eventually, their existences becomes one of self-imposed debility, to live out their time as carbon based machines whose sole purpose is to produce shit and piss. Dr. Reebs just broke the news that this guy didn't even make it through to the end of his mom's honeymoon.

BABY FAT

Labeling something as a miracle has become rhetoric. Does
imitation mayonnaise deserve such a moniker? Blueberries? How
about raw shrimp turned into suckling pig?

Sure, Albert and Kate were ecstatic that their boy was born
with two arms and two legs, two eyes, two ears, ten fingers and
toes. A symmetric baby is always a joy. Now several months
later, the child was still alive, with thicker wisps of blonde
hair, though he was still as bald as his father. He giggled
constantly, as if he knew life was as good as it probably could
ever get: suckling on mommy's teat for hours on end, getting
shit and piss cleaned up for him as soon as they exited his
body, and mommy and daddy constantly hovering as if they were
the Secret Service protecting the leader of the free world. The

baby only smelled of artificially constructed flavors of flowers, sweetly tart through the nose onto the tongue, made so by vigilant diaper checks and application and reapplications of every sort of over-advertised lotions and herbal butt pastes. Xander was born with a silver spoon in every orifice: Burberry onesies, cruising in the baby beemer Bugaboo, an ornate crib constructed of handcrafted Brazilian hardwood, mahogany chests overflowing with so many playthings as to seemingly allow for a different toy to be played with every hour of his waking infancy, a kitchen pantry stocked to look like the baby aisle at Whole Foods, and bookshelves stacked with worn copies of every latest bestselling parenting self-help book. He was fast on his way to a life of Perrier and pastel sweaters.

The way this baby's development was being curried, he should have already been well on his way to inventing a more efficient biofuel or curing breast cancer, but in all these visits to Albert and Kate's home, usually invited under the guise of a dinner party or a meaningless birthday though just a rouse for occasion to show off baby Xander, all I have ever seen that baby do is eat. Mom boasted that she nursed to near empty and still had to supplement with a fortune of formula to keep Xander happy. Dad beams of Xander going through baby food so fast as to require weekly grocery trips to replenish their

supply of mush filled glass jars in bulk lots. They were proud
of his consumptive abilities, as if imitating livestock was a
virtue. They scoffed at their pediatrician's advice to moderate
his intake, noting Xander's weight has always been off the
standard growth chart, and simply dismissed his skyrocketing
percentiles by repeating, "Babies were meant to grow and that's
just what he's doing. Xander is going to be a football player.
Hahaha!"

A baby's birth weight is normally supposed to double by
about 6 months, triple by 12 months. Xander was born 6 lbs. 4
oz. (the statistic widely known by most of Chicagoland from
being on Albert and Katie's *Baby Xander* mass email list) and now
at 9 months was about 25 lbs. Quadrupled size in 9 months. His
Escherichia coli like accelerated growth rate seemed at risk of
outpacing the expansion of this universe, until the margins of
his mass faded beyond our local supercluster. This baby had
become a crawling food dumpster.

It couldn't have helped that when mom was carrying Xander,
she went crazy with food. She was always a slender adult, from
a lifestyle of peer pressured restrictive dieting, but when she
got pregnant, she took it as a golden pass to eat anything she
wanted. No more granola and yogurt for breakfast; it was
McGriddles time. Low -fat turkey and swiss on whole wheat for

lunch? Try a double stack meal. Dinners of grilled salmon atop a garden salad with a glass of red wine turned to spooning into a quart of chocolate ice cream with Reeses Pieces mashed into it. She gained fifty pounds – fifty pounds to kick out a kid that weighed about seven. Everyone excuses weight gain in lieu of pregnancy, so when that dam of social deprivation finally cracks from sperm fertilizing egg, it unleashes burgers, fries and chocolate shakes. Because of Kate, Xander had been awash in calories since he was a few cells old.

His abnormal weight development pushed me to cycle through unlikely differentials of congenital anomalies like Prader-Willi or Bardet-Biedl and refer him to a pediatric endocrinologist in case of some hormonal disorder, but those were CYA workups, as he was developing normally in every other way. The most memorable quote from the endocrinologist's consultation letter: "Although his weight gain is unusually accelerated, I do not suspect it is due to anything other than a robust appetite and overfeeding."

Now when he comes into my office for his well-child checkups, it is a misnomer – he is far from well. His parents appear to be force feeding him as if getting a goose ready for the foie-gras harvest. Then they ask me to assess his development. He was only developing how a rancher would

7

describe his steers as developing. Then they have the gall to
rush him into the office in full panic with an emergency of
"spitting up". Imagine if you force fed yourself a family-sized
pan of al fredo? Re-tasting that creamy regurgitation? How
about getting a hose rammed down your throat and a tanker of
milk getting unloaded into you? This baby was not
pathologically vomiting with a bowel obstruction or at risk of
starvation from spitting up too much of his meals; he was just
trying to normalize his intake by gurgling up some extra milk.
Spitting up was this baby's only recourse.

I remember at one month of age, Kate was concerned that he
wasn't eating a much as usual. Xander had previously fed on
each breast for fifteen minutes each, then took four to six
ounces of formula every three hours on top of that; Kate was
worried at the visit because even though he was still on each
breast for fifteen minutes, he only wanted two to three ounces
of formula afterward. She thought he was wasting away. I
remember I had seen him the week before for some bogus
constipation complaint from Kate (expelling normal stools "only"
twice a day is not abnormal) and he had weighed nine pounds, six
ounces. Today, he weighed ten pounds, six ounces: a weight gain
of one pound in just one week. A normal one month old should be
gaining about an ounce a day - Xander was filling his cells at

more than double that rate. The kid wasn't eating as much now because he was simply stuffed. Kate was so used to seeing Xander put away superhuman amounts of milk that when he finally scaled back his intake due to constant over-satiety, she thought he was sick. I guess he was sick, with food.

Maybe there is no such thing as an excessively fat baby. That is, no baby should go on a diet, no baby should do South Beach, and no baby should have to worry about getting in bathing suit shape. But Xander is making me reconsider, because this is one fat ass baby. Look at this kid squiggle in his Stokke Sleepi crib. The crib's joists are creaking under the shearing strain. He has rolls of baby fat insulating a Buddha body supporting a candy-apple melon. He looks like the less hairy twin of the overstuffed Vermont stuffed teddy bear plopped down at the head of his crib. The bear's thread face had the appearance of someone watching a fat man down a dozen deep fried bacon wrapped butter sticks. Most stuffed bears have the same face of naive, saccharine optimism as the Snuggle bear, but this one had an abject look of disgust from thinking this fat baby wasn't going to make it to his next birthday because of a heart attack. The bear's eyes seemed enraged at the sight of his de-conditioned bedmate, with its furry body language stiffened in aggressive posturing to say, "Hey baby, what the hell have you been eating? Why are you so damn fat? I'm a pear shaped fur ball of hibernation storage, and even I think you look disgustingly huge. Ever hear of saying you're full? Passing on seconds? And get your ass crawling on a treadmill sometimes. Those legs were made for moving, not storing blubber. Geez."

And here I was for this kid's nine month "birthday" party.

"Ooh, Dr. Grant, do you want to hold Xander? Just sit there on the rocking chair, it's a Dutailier Glider," Kate squealed as she plopped Xander onto me.

Great, now I have Xander on my lap cutting blood flow to my lower legs while having to listen to him gasp for air in between feeding himself handfuls of Cheerios. The kid had a kangaroo-like pouch sewn onto the front of his overalls that was just holding Cheerios. Now that Xander had officially started junior foods, he was likely feeding on mounds of Cheerios and soft veggies that would easily compete with his parent's dinner portions. My leg was in tingling pain from Xander's body weight tourniquet. At least it was an amazing rocking chair. Wish I had one to sit in just to watch football. There were three in this living room alone.

"I bet you haven't held him since you delivered him."

The clowns surrounding the Xander show starting piping in with their usual interjections:

"Look at that, he's feeding himself!"

"Let's take a picture!"

"Smile, Dr. Grant, smile, cheeeese!"

All that I could muster in this photo with this ugly baby was the uglier baby of my gritting teeth and my every facial muscle straining to forcibly upturn the corners of my mouth. My forearms were burning trying to hold this kid steady. Why are they trying to take these pictures with a small, handheld camera? Pictures of this baby are going to need at least three sequential pictures taken with a real good SLR and collaged together, because a shot from a satellite is the only thing that has a chance of capturing this kid in a single snap. A dozen other members of the watching gallery start to applaud and coo at the awful picture of me holding the baby, and their excitement plays sarcastic in my mind and I let a few chuckles escape, but when I closer examine everyone's faces, most look to be genuinely excited with the results of the camera work. They must be great actors because no one should be this pleased with a snapshot of a lanky nerd balancing a squirming piglet on his knee.

I always knew that in coming back to my hometown to practice pediatrics, I risked having to care for the kids of some familiar faces. I went to high school with half of the faces in this room. But in caring for Albert and Kate's only kid, they had erased the boundary between doctor and patient, and instead I became just another member of their family. Hell, here I am at a made up birthday milestone, posing with him for the family and friend paparazzi.

I eventually pass Xander down the line to some more eager arms, having to audibly grunt and conjure up every bit of my bicep strength to pick him up to make the handoff, and then I got up to stand at the outskirts of the living room and kitchen. Look at that kitchen. Boxes of bulk Cheerios and organic baby food stacked against the wall. I turn and look out the window to the driveway curbside and I see reams of flattened food boxes lying on the grass waiting to be taken by garbage men, who no doubt wonder to themselves when this couple had quadruplets.

Albert and Kate actually did have twins, and Xander was the larger; so large as to have literally consumed the life out of his twin brother.

The preciousness of a lone survivor is rewarded with the spoils meant for two. "A miracle", always say mom and dad, "a miracle that Xander survived", in between kisses from forehead to toe, "A miracle he's how he is now." Awwws and sniffles and tearing. My eyes were tearing from the effort of quelling down bubbling vomit.

When Xander came out of mom, he was large, limp and flushed. He looked like a piece of raw jumbo shrimp. His body was struggling to adapt to the influx of too much blood, stolen from his womb-mate via vascular malformations. He spent weeks in intensive care getting his hematocrit normalized with exchange transfusions of saline for blood before being brought home. His brother subsequently came out small, limp and blue. Raw escargot. His brother spent days in intensive care trying to get his hematocrit normalized with series of blood transfusions and died from complications of severe anemia, the heart eventually failing to pump his thinned blood to all the vital organs of his body. If you had placed them side to side at the time of death, Xander looked as if he was a few Russian nesting dolls removed from un-encasing his brother.

There was a clear winner of that shared womb. Even with the multiple attempts by doctors to level the field with amnioreduction and foetoscopic laser treatments while they were both in-utero, only one survived. Xander was a pure consumer, and in the most basic Darwinian struggle, he had consumed his way to victory. Though, he did almost kill himself by consuming too much, but maybe that was worth the risk to ensure he won. A lesson already ingrained in the womb: whoever consumes the most, wins by the most.

Now, Xander appears to want to become the last man on earth by out-consuming the rest of the world.

Party break time. My temples were pounding, and my body felt weak from the strain of feigning fun. Sneaking into the back hallway, I just plopped down onto the carpet right across from the bathroom. If anyone finds me I can dismiss my absence with saying I drank too much coffee or that the pound of birthday cake they force-fed me was just not sitting right. I peeked around the corner into the baby's room. All DaVinci furniture. A cherry wood changing table. A BOB jogger tucked in the corner. The room looked much smaller than its actual square footage, space being shrunk by a swing, a play center, chests of toys, every species of stuffed animal, enough picture books stacked into a bookcase to illustrate the history of the Earth, boxes of chlorine free diapers and wipes in gross, and a 50-inch flat screen television mounted on the ceiling above the crib playing baby stimulating nonsense on a loop.

A toilet flushed. I scrambled to my feet just as the bathroom door swings open. Albert.

He jumps aback. "Hey, geez, you scared me."

"Sorry, Al. Just waiting. Too much birthday cake."

"Me too. You having fun?"

"Of course. I always have fun. Xander is really growing up."

"Yeah, he sure is."

A beam of sunlight from the hallway window caught Albert's face and betrayed drying watery streaks.

"Hey Al what's with your eyes?"

Rubbing, "What? No. Just made a birthday cake deposit in there. Way too much cake and coffee. I'll let you get to it then, too."

Albert smiled and scooted past me back to the party. I guess I'll have to go into the bathroom to continue my break.

I grab a seat onto the furry blue covered toilet seat. It's impeccably clean in here. And smells just like Xander. I expected at least a waft of week old possum, but whatever went on before I got here, it was long dissipated. Even the diaper genie smelled flowery. A bag of old baby shit smeared on cloth and plastic had been made to have no hint of mustiness, methane or acridity. That is until I threw up into the bathtub. Way too much cake and coffee.

I turn on the bath faucet for a second to wash down the brown and black, and then take a Kleenex to wipe my mouth. The trash is overflowing with freshly used Kleenex. If it was any other guy in here before me, I would've assumed they were jizz rags. But this had been Albert. Never a smudge, from prep school to college to fatherhood, from lacrosse team captain to crew team captain to his own law practice, from home to church to home to church. This was not the guy that would take a break from his own son's birthday party to tug one out in the bathroom to a copy of *Marie Claire*. These were tear rags. Why did this guy steal away to cry alone in the bathroom?

Married too early, kid too early, and the kid carrying your name is a load. Every stage in life should've been an improvement from the last, and it had been, until now. Imagine the long-awaited fruit of finding a worthy mate, years of financial preparation, months of living by ovulation cycles, and forty weeks of careful care being a excrement factory of a butterball turkey with your surname on the birth certificate. Life was less a Church of Latter Day Saints commercial and more a focus of pumping food into a never-satiated mouth so it can make more shit and piss to clear away. Crying alone in the bathroom was a no-brainer.

I walked out of the bathroom, stomach getting queasier as I hear the white noise chatter, then hear a higher pitch of suckling noises coming from Xander's bedroom. The door is cracked open just a bit.

Imagine a breast engorged so that it has grown proportionally larger and voluptuous, not in an artificial implant forced rise or in an obesity related flop forward, but in the way of fantastic genetics -- natural fullness held into impossibly high soft mounds by only the elasticity of its own skin, with mousse-whipped delicate cafe-au-lait centers pointing directly at you. Then imagine a pale pot bellied pig gnawing at the teat. Suckling pig never sounded so unappetizing. I expected the breast to deflate, making the slow flubbering of a dying balloon. The electricity of discovering partial nudity dispersed into the ground rod as if grandma had suddenly walked into the scene. Xander was ruining breasts. Perfect breasts.

He was ruining lives. Dad was already broken. And in the privacy of Xander's room, Kate dropped the glow of party host and settled in to show her fatigue. A graying forelock seemed more apparent, her shoulders sagged, and she was fighting sleep as she was feeding Xander. His occasional biting was the only thing keeping her awake. I'm sure she wishes she could bite that baby back. Or bite her boobs off and slowly bleed out. Or go back a year and bite off Al's member so it couldn't have pumped in the seed that fertilized her egg. Or go back and decide not to marry the first guy after breaking up with a longtime boyfriend. Or not decide to get pregnant during year

one of marriage. She used to love traveling and indulging her
inner foodie -- she once blew an entire semester's book money on
a four star bender of haute cuisine -- but now she was just a
feedbag, a vessel for providing breast milk. Her eagerness to
speed into motherhood must now feel like a sow galloping to the
slaughterhouse.

She started to stir back from her wink of a nap. She
looked towards the door.

I shuffled back to the party. Al was chitchatting with
some big-haired grandma in between bites of cake, everyone was
picking through heaping plates of buffet in between open mouthed
bursts of laughter revealing partially masticated gobs of food
on teeth, and new guests were continually arriving with their
crock pots of foodstuff to replenish the buffet line. No New
Testament Jesus miracle needed here to feed thousands, just a
one liner at the bottom of the invite: "Potluck lunch."

I just kept walking, slipping unnoticed out the door. My
car was blocked in by a Mercedes SUV. I just took a sharp left
turn through the lawn, clipping an inflatable blue bear, and
jarred over the curb onto the side street, and pressed the gas.
I got home rather quick. I slept the rest of the day
uninterrupted. Food coma.

MILK MONSTER

Xander's finally here for his two year old well child
checkup. I've been really looking forward to this. After
today, I only have to schedule that kid once a year for
checkups. His first year was rough – scheduled visits at one,
two, four, six, nine and twelve months of age. The second year
forward was better, but still too many times – visits at fifteen
and eighteen months, and now at two years old. That was eight
scheduled visits no matter if Xander stayed completely healthy.
But unfortunately, that eight was only on top of all the other
bullshit "emergency" clinic visits – Kate accidently giving him
Tylenol three and a half hours apart instead of the recommended
four, a 1x1 centimeter rash that was here the previous day but
not visible the day of the visit but still needing diagnosis,
and the numerous times he had a "fever" of 98.6 degrees because

of a parent-diagnosed condition of a lower than normal baseline temperature of 96 degrees. These well child visits were painful, as Albert and Kate used the visits as opportunity for an exposition on the minutiae of Xander. This two year old visit did not offer anything new: a relatively healthy kid with an accompanying rambling monologue describing every hiccup and fart as possible proof why he might not be well. At least it was just Kate with Xander this time.

"Yesterday, Xander ate ten chicken McNuggets and a handful of fries, but then only drank half a glass of milk, so I got real worried that he just didn't drink enough for all that salt, so I really pushed the fruit juice and Pedialyte for the next three hours, but then he threw up all his food, so then I thought he might have lost all of his lunch and might be getting malnourished, so I gave him a bowl of macaroni and cheese with some apple juice, but he threw that up too, so I think he has some sort of stomach bug, so can I get an antibiotic, Dr. Grant?

"First off, I don't think he's sick. I think he just ate way too much. Secondly…"

"But Dr. Grant, he eats that much pretty much every day and rarely vomits. I mean, if he eats too much every day, why is his weight normal?"

"His weight is not normal. Look at his growth chart here.
The points are barely within the boundaries of the paper. He
hasn't fit inside of the normal curve since he was two months
old."

"But that's just his normal curve, his own special curve,
above all the other curves. And he needs to eat to keep up with
his full growth potential. Right now, he just needs an
antibiotic to get over this stomach bug. I don't want him to
get so sick he loses weight."

"He threw up all that food because he ate too much; I would
barely be able put down a full burger and fries with a glass of
whole milk, much less then to chase it with a quart of juice and
a half pound of macaroni. His weight is abnormally high for a
baby his age because he eats way too much. And he eats way too
much McDonald's."

"Oh, but he loves it. Maybe the McDonald's gave him the
stomach bug? Or food poisoning! Now that I think about it, we
did go to one we don't normally go to. It was on the South
Side."

"Xander does not have a stomach bug or food poisoning."

"Could we get an antibiotic just in case?"

"Even if he did have a stomach bug, most stomach bugs are
viruses and as I have told you many, many times before,

antibiotics don't kill viruses. And even by some bizarre
happenstance, if he did have some bacterial stomach bug, even
with most bacterial gastrointestinal infections, we wouldn't use
antibiotics anyway. Especially in someone that looks as good as
he does right now." Xander was now literally hanging off the
exam table with just his arms, panting and trying to do mini
pull-ups. "In any case, he does not have any infection, he
just ate too much."

"Well, we're going to a buffet with his grandparents for
dinner, so we'll see if he can eat his usual plates. If he
can't, I'll just call the answering service later and maybe you
can call something in for him."

And it goes on like that for another twenty minutes; twenty
more minutes of waste before getting down to any of the physical
exam or anticipatory guidance issues. His weight gain is again
ridiculous today; another plot point well above the boundaries
of the standard curve, exponentially continuing its rise. I had
to hand-draw an extension of the graphing lines onto the top of
the paper just to plot Xander today. The kid has a quadruple
chin. He looked like baby Sumo in just his mawashi. A two year
old should be scampering around the room, getting into the box
of exam gloves on the wall or peering under the flip lid of the
garbage can or mussing the pile of picture books on the side

table, but Xander was slowly lumbering around the room sucking on a sippy-cup of milk. And at this visit, he looked a bit pale.

"How much milk does he drink, Kate?

"We finish a gallon every one or two days."

I know Albert and Kate don't like the taste of milk so that "we" is really just a "he".

"That is way too much milk for him."

"He loves it, and would drink it all day if he could. So we let him because milk is healthy, right?"

Milk is a great food, but like everything, in moderation. Carrots are great, but if that's all you eat, you'll wither away as your skin turns starkly orange. Literally die looking like a carrot. Xander's problem with milk is simple science. Red blood cells need iron to function. Milk is not that great a source of usable iron. It's tough to get iron otherwise when milk is being abused as the major part of an unbalanced diet, so dark vegetables and lean red meats become an afterthought. This kid just drank himself to iron-deficiency anemia. Here's a two year old kid already causing health problems by overconsumption of food - a milk monster. And he has a sippy-cup in his hands right now, sucking back on that white as if he were a man with a breast shaped mug filled with beer.

"In moderation, Kate, you have to only let him drink milk in moderation. You have to cut his entire diet into one of moderation or he's going to get unhealthy, er, unhealthier."

I think back on the history of his office visits, when I initially gave just gentle suggestions that Xander was a bit chubby, and then started stating the kid was fat, and then just telling Albert and Kate to stop feeding their roly-poly so damn much. Now here we are at two years of age and my words have dented them as much as a bullet into Superman. Maybe today I should show Kate a picture of what I see is up the road for Xander: his head pasted on a nude Rosie O'Donnell.

During many of Kate's office ramblings, I often day-dreamt about calling DCFS, reporting abuse via over-feeding, or in the least claim neglect of health, but ultimately, has any kid ever been taken away from his parents due to the kid being too fat? Neglect is not feeding your kid; it is not feeding your kid too much, right? Maybe if I had gotten the process started early, Xander vs. the State of Illinois could have become a landmark case, maybe the next Scopes monkey trial, the next Roe vs. Wade. But the only open case going on right now was Xander vs. Milk, and Xander was absolutely winning.

Albert and Kate always had the same response: "Oh, he'll grow out of it." Deluded ridiculousness. Fat is not a pair of

OshKosh B'Gosh overalls. Body rolls and extra breasts are not like pubertal acne. The only thing Xander is growing out of is being able to externally verify his sex as his penis is fast disappearing into his pubic fat pad. Instead of just being a fat little kid, he's going to become a fat grade-schooler, a fat teen, a fat adult and a fat-ass corpse. Let's say best case scenario he becomes tall like his dad - he'll just be a tall fat guy that may be able to create an optical illusion with his height that he's only obese and not morbidly obese.

I had the nurse do a fingerstick hemoglobin. Xander didn't make a peep as she got a drop of blood from his fingertip. I half expected the blood to be milkshake thick with chunks of fat globules, but it was a normal runny red. Xander seemed oddly interested in the whole procedure, and was ecstatic about the SpongeBob Band-Aid. His hemoglobin was 9.4. This aspect of being a doctor must be like being a homicide detective: in pursuit of solving a case, the only true consistent discovery is the disappointment in humanity.

"You really let Xander drink that much milk?"

"Sure, why not?"

Maybe I'll try a series of simple sentences this time.

"Xander is anemic from drinking too much milk. He can get really sick if you let him drink that much. All that juice is not helping, either. He's drinking way too many calories. He's ridiculously overweight."

"Oh, Dr. Grant, you're such a worrier. I'll try to cut down on his milk. As for his weight, I am sure he'll just grow out of it. He's just going to be our little football player!"

Fuck.

THE WHITE WHALE

Albert and Kate have been inviting me out to dinner for
months, and I have been skillfully dodging them with excuses of
being a too busy doctor. The last time I saw Xander was when
Kate rushed him into the office for a cold last winter. "He's
just got a cold, Kate." "But he has a cough, runny nose and
fever." "That's a cold, Kate." You can tell a lot about a
parent as to when during the normal 7-10 day course of a cold,
they bring their kid in to see the doctor. Some rush their kid
in after mere hours of symptoms, as if the standard cold
symptoms were the tip of some life-threatening illness - telling
of overprotective and over-bearing helicopter parents, or people
with bags of rocks for brains. Some parents wait until about
day 3, when a cold's symptoms typically are at their worst,
again attributing the normal worsening and persistent symptoms

of a typical cold as some harbinger of death - jumpy and paranoid parents, but better than the overprotective and overbearing, though very much still that their brains are bags of rocks as well. Both types of parents are bringing in their kids with the expectation of some antibiotic, not understanding the uselessness of antibiotics in treating viral illnesses, and carrying senses of entitlement that every boogery nose needs instant meds on meds, regardless of efficacy, because they as parents somehow knows more medicine than everyone else. Why did I waste my years on college, med school, internship, residency and years of private practice when all I needed to learn medicine was to have a kid and be able to Google a list of symptoms? Then there are the parents that don't bring their kids into the doctor's office for simple colds, parents that know what a cold looks like, remembers what a cold feels like (as everyone has had a cold before), and just takes care of their kids with home care until they improve in 7-10 days. As a result, smart and sensible parents like that are unfortunately the ones that I don't get to see too much. Kate brought Xander in that day after 2 hours of runny nose and fever. Thankfully I've been able to avoid them since. But because of the seemingly never ending requirement of Continuing Medical Education to keep my licensure up to date, I go to Wisconsin

Dells for a conference and decide to eat at the hotel's restaurant for dinner instead of ordering room service and catching Bulls vs. Bucks on TV.

I was just waiting for my table. Damn fifteen minute wait for this dinosaur themed restaurant. The triceratops robot nodding at the front door was taunting me. It appeared to start shouting my name.

"Dr. Grant! Dr. Grant!" The voice was ricocheting off the robot and not coming out of its jaws. "Dr. Grant! It's me Xander!"

The kid came running at a full sprint up to me, every foot strike sounding like it was breaking tile. He had a King-sized Hershey bar in paw and his face was smeared in chocolate. He was in swimming trunks and a slightly wet white T-shirt clinging to his rolls. At least he ran the few dozen feet to me and burned off about a dozen calories.

Kate came up just behind him.

"Hi, Dr. Grant, crazy seeing you here!"

"Hi, Kate, what are you guys doing here?"

"Just a quick weekend at the water parks up here, Xander loves the water, he's like a fish."

He obviously looked more like a whale. A small one, but still a whale. No way was he resembled any type of fish. Maybe she meant fish in the colloquial use as referring to any sea creature as a fish.

"Where's Albert?"

"He's meeting us here tomorrow, after he gets off work. What are you doing here?"

"Just here at this cardiology conference until tomorrow."

"Are you here by yourself?"

"Yeah, sure am. These conferences are a great opportunity for me to get away for some alone time."

Except when I run into patients. It feels like when as a kid I would run into teachers running errands. Breaking away from set roles in routine settings gets weird. It's always a bit awkward going to the neighborhood Portillo's Hot Dogs and running into the parents and the seven year old kid who was just at the office with such bad constipation and withholding that he crapped his pants during the peristalsis release of the rectal exam, and then watching him eat nothing but cheese fries when I just gave the parents a lecture on how they needed to up his fiber intake and try to cut down on cheese and starch. Or the mom that is now stuffing her giggling one year old with handfuls of McDonald's who had just rushed her daughter into my office without an appointment spouting off loudly in the waiting room about some mystery life-threatening illness that had symptoms of poor eating and a "fever" of 99.2 lasting an hour, and then spending the entire visit demanding antibiotics to cure her baby lest her baby become more lethargic without some emergent treatment. Or running into the fattest patient in my practice a few hundred miles away at a Midwest version of a Vegas hotel, and then getting a live show of him erasing chocolate.

"Why don't you join us for dinner here then? I know Xander will love it."

Then right on cure, Xander popped the rest of his candy bar into his mouth and piped up, "Yeah! Please, Dr. Grant? I'll teach you how to draw a stegosaurus."

Even an overly chubby kid's cocoa-smeared, moon-faced smile was impossible for me to shoot down. So here I am being seated in a booth in the shape of a brontosaurus, across from Xander and Kate, about to spend the next few hours eating dinner with them and learning about all things Xander. Time needed to bleed out quickly, and awkward silences would only prolong the pain. I started by asking a question I knew would kill at least half-an-hour without much of my participation: "So, how's Xander been?"

So Kate went on about how much he could read now and all the activities she had signed him up for and how he was going to kindergarten in the fall and how great a kid he was. I could

tune out her voice easily, just as I could tune out dozens of
wailing babies in a nursery as I focused on examining just one,
but now my focus was being steered to using my peripherals to
examine two other types of babies. I must have always had my
nose buried in Xander's chart during Kate's ramblings at his
office visits, and Kate must have dressed conservatively at
those visits, and the sourness that descended onto my
disposition in anticipation of Xander's office visits must have
also put pause to my manhood, because now I couldn't stop
looking at her somethings. To me, Kate was not classically
beautiful, a little too much forehead for that, but she did have
two assets that must have contributed to Xander downing breast
milk in such quantities when he was a baby. And she had them in
full on display in her bikini with her cover-up only partially
covering them up. And it was sharply cold in the restaurant. I
was surprised at my maleness for continuing to glance at them,
knowing on whom they were attached. They were softened from
time, but still supple and ample with just barely a noticeable
sag. And the cleavage was wonderfully tight in its spacing, not
artificially mashed together as with a push up bra or bizarrely
frog-eyed like the implant variety.

"Look, Dr. Grant, I drew a Stegasaurus!"

Xander was furiously scribbling onto his placemat with a green crayola. His shirt was still wet. He actually had a large pair showing as well. They were floppy buds, as if he were an obese preadolescent girl, but they were ample enough to fit the definition of breasts. A five year old boy with a chest like a fudge-loving, never exercising preteen.

The waitress came and we placed our orders. Me and Xander ordered the same meatloaf dinner - called the Stegasaurus Loaf here. Kate ordered the T-Rex burger platter which was just a standard bacon cheeseburger with waffle fries. She must work out quite a bit to stay in the shape she's currently in whilst eating bacon, grilled ground beef and deep fried crisscrosses of potato. Or maybe she's just eating her one bad meal allotment for this week. Or maybe she's just splurging on these calories because she's on vacation.

Now I sound like one of them, where the current obesity generating lifestyle is rationalized as just a temporary hiatus to the healthier lifestyle which will start after coming back from vacation, or after the holidays, or in the New Year, or after this birthday, or in the summer - always about to start at some never-arriving, ever-delayed future. Where massive volumes of food go in, massive volumes of excuses burp out. All that needs to be said to complete the classic rhetoric is to go on about the exploits of the skinnier, fitter person of the long ago past that could've beat anyone in physical feats of strength and stamina, and then complain about the various current joint aches and resultant immobility that is preventing proper exercise in between bites of a fast disappearing Philly cheesesteak with whiz. The common path of mental self-preservation seems to be to gloss over the current state of deconditioning by shifting focus to a future change, and then try to impose an image of potential fitness with tales of the unverifiable past.

Oh good, the food is here. I was starving. Look at this Stegosaurus loaf. The waitress needed two arms to unload it from the standing tray. Restaurants seem to pack a garbage can with food, then flip it over onto a plate as a means to measure a single portion, and The Dinostaurant was no different. How am I supposed to eat all of this? Purge halfway through my dinner into the porcelain Velociraptor head in the bathroom? I guess the restaurants are only giving people what they want, only doing what they need to do in order to keep people waddling into here, as opposed to there, where the mound of mashed potatoes down the street is only chest high as opposed to head high here. Though looking around the restaurant, it looks like most of the people dining would say that this was an appropriate portion for

one. The three hundred pound bearded guy seated next to our
table just got up from his booth with a grunt, and all that was
left on his table was a plate of chicken wing bones, a platter
with steak gristle aside a few smears of mashed potatoes, a
saucer with a shallow puddle of melted ice cream and chocolate
syrup, and three empty beer bottles. It seems what people want
to do at restaurants is to gorge and gorge on three thousand
calorie meals in a race to over-satiety. It is as if the
primitive biologic urge to store calories that existed during
man's times of food scarcity has only accelerated as food has
gotten more abundant. Everyone seems to be storing fat for some
Armageddeon. It is an entirely American concept, though. I
cannot think of another worldly cuisine where the serving plate
is so large, and sits underneath a mound of meat with a just
sprinkling of vegetables. Plates are undeniably smaller
everywhere else in the world, and meat is used more as a garnish
than as the meal entire. Most have to get by with what we would
consider weeds and bugs, spending most of their days procuring
and protecting their non-guaranteed meals. Food here is an
entitlement in excess. It must be offensively odd for others to
watch the average American at a buffet -- plates overfilled with
food, much of it going uneaten and cleared from the table as a
routine into the waste bins of busboys. It is no accident that

the domestic health perils of obesity, like heart disease and
diabetes, start developing in new immigrants from cultures
traditionally without those ills, a result of their increasing
assimilation to their new homeland's cuisine. And those
conditions continue on in their proceeding generations as their
plates grow more American with every bite. Looks like the food
arriving to the table had created a natural pause to Kate's
update. Damn. The food just got here. This is no time to sit
in silence. Better rev back up her train of thought.

"Sounds like he's doing great, what else have you guys been
up to?"

This dinosaur shaped meatloaf was comically large but
admittedly delicious – soft and moist, seasoned lightly with
thyme and topped with a tangy sweet tomato based glaze. The
mashed potatoes were fork-drippy creamy, as if they were more
butter than potato. This was going down so smooth that, for a
second, I envied the heavies that ate like this every meal and
got to enjoy more quantity of this goodness. This place was an
assembly line for the obese. They were filing in through the
restaurant's front entrance, advancing to their seats crabby and
antsy, lumbering to have kilocalories added to body at every
course, and exiting out patting bellies and burping. And in a
curious stroke of hotel planning, at the exit everyone had to

trundle right past the hotel's fitness center, situated behind
full length windows across the causeway of the restaurant.
Large glass fronted lonely treadmills and ellipticals,
resistance machines were noticeably dusty and the free-weights
looked rusty - this was a microcosm in the battle for fat.
Super-size portions at every restaurant, candy and chocolate at
every checkout counter begging for that impulse buy, and
portions becoming so outsized that eating a foot-long sandwich
becomes the "healthier" choice; salad and yogurt choices placed
alongside those Super-sizers, gyms hanging bright banners
advertising discounted memberships at every corner, bookstores
with shelves and shelves of fad diets.   In that battle of good
and evil, good always wins, as in what feels good going down the
hatch.

This meatloaf is really good but I can't finish it. Xander
had already long cleaned his plate.

The rest of dinner was blur of vacation tales to Disney
World and grandma's house in Arizona, and of cleavage, both in a
pert female and saggy boy variety.

Dessert? Pass for me. I doubt I will be hungry again
until late afternoon tomorrow. Xander begged for and got a
chocolate sundae with the works.

Yes, the dinner check, the official end to dinner out. The
dinner check is also a time for reflection, to think about the
cost of the evening. Encased in a faux-leather sheath, it is a
chronicling of the events of the last hour -- appetizers,
drinks, main courses, desserts. How much did it cost to become
full? How many rounds of food did it take to be full? After
all this, am I even full? The number next to the food item is
the final dollar calculation of providing all this consumption:
finding suitable land, buying the land, clearing the land,
tilling the land, planting the land, fertilizing the land,
watering and watering and watering, harvesting, processing,
packaging, transporting, gassing up, transporting some more,
opening a restaurant, advertising the restaurant, hiring chef
talent, hiring hosts and servers, lighting stoves and ovens,
buying the food, cooking the food, presenting the food, serving
the food and finally finding someone to eat the food. Today,
the dollar cost of all that effort was a little over $50. The
real life cost was growing a fat kid a little fatter, and
snipping more time from the end. For me, it would be more
appropriate if the check came inside a barf-bag. I had eaten
way too much. Fifty bucks must be the going rate at the
Dinostaurant to feel like yakking.

Xander ordered the same meatloaf dinner as I did, and he was leaving his plate clean. I had a third of my loaf and mashed potatoes in a doggy bag and felt sick. And I didn't have a Hershey bar aperitif or a chocolate sundae finisher. The puzzled inquiries from obese patients as to why they are obese are always deluded, as essentially they're insinuating, "*I'm doing everything I can and yet I'm still paradoxically fat.*" The reason is child placemat puzzle simple. Pick any aspect of your diet and there's the answer. Three meals of charger plate-sized portions every day, or snacking on the many versions of sugared butter in between each of those meals, or washing it all down with gallons of juice and soda, or taking in more calories in one meal than seconds of cardio over the entire day?

I picked up the check, thanked Kate for her company, and excused myself with a comment of an early start in the morning. Xander gave me a hug around the leg.

Great. Now my khakis smell like chlorine and there are probably chocolate handprints behind my knee. But at least I was finally going back to my room. I was looking forward to sleeping off this bomb I just ate, but not looking forward to tonight's probable dream. My subconscious had just been flooded with food, breasts and near vomiting. What can come out of that mix?

Probably something along the lines of an M&M ejaculating chocolate syrup onto bare breasts. I'm going to skip the continental breakfast tomorrow morning.

THE FAT KID IN CLASS

I've seen this coming for a long time.

Fat little babies and chubby toddlers have little real
world consequences while they wallow in calories in front of
their parents' eyes. They might even be considered cute rolys.
But once they hit school and are around other kids, it's a
different story. Kids are cruel.

Picking on the fat kid is childhood's oldest sport. It's
history reaches deep: imagine the strained grunts when a fat
cavekid struggled up a rock hill with all his cavemates already
gleefully at the top, then the grunting laughter as Chunky
Caveboy slipped and tumbled back down to the base, or the
embarrassment when a fat Athenian kid bent over to pick up a
stone ball and ripped his toga to bare ass, or Lil' Tubby never

being picked to play kick the can because he has never been able twenty-two skidoo fast enough or long enough to kick any can.

Xander's problems really started around the time of his first grade physical.

"Dr. Grant, Xander is really having a tough time at school."

For the first time, Xander was quiet in the exam room, seated on a stool, playing a GameBoy. No more manic puppy dog exuberance, rather, he was just a sluggish hippo wading in mudwater to avoid the midday sun.

"What's going on in school?"

"He says he doesn't like it. And he doesn't want to go outside and play. He just sits around and watches TV or plays video games."

It's a common complaint with this generation of kids. When Kate and I were growing up in the old neighborhood, all we did was play outside: baseball in the summer, basketball in the fall, football in the snow. We could spend hours throwing rocks at a tree stump or playing Marco Polo in the pool at her house. The only kids we didn't know in the neighborhood were the pale, overweight home-schooled kids that got tired too quickly for any sport and always just wanted to bike to 7-Eleven to get Slurpees and Snickers. We got those kids to stop hanging out with us

real quick using the simplest of methods: "Beat it, lardbutt".
Nowadays, kicking out the fat kid from play would mean
dissolving whole neighborhoods.

"Dr. Grant, I think it's because Xander is shy."

Shy of what, two hundred pounds? How can she not see
what's going on here? She must be too close to the fat. Like
when my fat grandmother would hug me when I was a kid and bury
my face in her belly's cavernous muffintop -- I could barely
breathe much less know what the hell was going on around me. I
guess Kate needs to hear it straight out of Xander.

"Xander, what's going on at school, little buddy?"

"Nothing."

"Are kids picking on you?"

Silence. Kate chimes in firmly, "Xander, Dr. Grant asked
you a question."

"Yeah, kids are picking on me."

It's no wonder. Xander is big. Kate is tall, slender
and in a cashmere turtleneck, wool dress pants and leather boots
today, and I am betting six year old Xander weighs as much as
she does right now, even with all of her fall clothing.

"Kate, you and I both know kids can be cruel, so it's just
one more reason to get Xander in better shape before the kids
really get mean."

"You're so right, Dr. Grant, I guess Xander just got sucked into this national childhood obesity crisis. Did you see Dateline last night? It's really a problem."

So a growing collection of fat kids are what constitutes an epidemic nowadays, a national crisis? It is an epidemic and crisis as much as credit card debt is an epidemic and two pack-a-day smokers dying of lung cancer is a crisis. It has become common culture to be overweight and the minutiae of how and why or who's responsible has become background noise. The collective of obese has become its own entity, separate from the individual gluttons that comprise it, effectively shifting the mindset of responsibility from person to some sweeping crisis. The Cuban Missile Crisis was a crisis, the beginnings of HIV was a crisis, kids going hungry is a crisis; kids eating double bacon cheeseburgers, large fries, and chocolate milkshakes every day is not a crisis. It is just simple overconsumption. The elephant in the room needs a bigger spotlight.

"What do you feed Xander, Kate?"

"Oh, a pretty balanced diet. He loves chicken and I always serve some vegetable with his meals. He loves fruit."

She said it as if Xander was just eating three ounces of grilled chicken with a small side salad and an apple every meal. As if he had grown wider because of a diet of lean protein,

fresh vegetables and fruit. No one has ever become morbidly
obese eating a balanced diet in proper portions. No one. The
evidence of poor dietary constitution is in the constitution of
double chins, accordion folding bellies and an appearance of
perpetual unisex pregnancy. Parents are always going to gloss
over the bad reality, either with doublespeak or outright lies,
to deflect any suggestion of their negligence or their child's
shortcomings.

"Chicken or chicken nuggets?"

"Chicken nuggets, I guess."

"And potato for a vegetable most of the time, right?"

"Oh, come on, Dr. Grant, it's not only potatoes. He likes
corn too."

"French fries and creamed corn?"

"Sometimes."

"And fruit cocktail or fruit roll-ups?"

"I guess both usually. I admit it, yes, he likes to eat
some junk, but he likes good food, too."

"Give me just one, and I will be one happy doctor."

"He loves broccoli."

"Really? Broccoli and what?"

"Are you talking about cheese? Because how can you eat
broccoli without cheese? That would just be wrong. Broccoli

doesn't taste too good on its own. Cheese is part of the food pyramid, isn't it?"

"Does he take seconds?"

"No, only usually at dinner. And I guess it would be considered seconds at breakfast too because sometimes he'll sneak a few extra pancakes at breakfast. But it is his favorite food. I swear, Xander would eat nothing but pancakes if we let him. But we try to push blueberry pancakes, though, for the fruit."

Then she smiled proudly, as if I should have written into the newspapers to alert them about this bit of ingenuity. Smiling about pushing fruit in the form of sprinkling dots of berry into pan fried cake batter drenched in maple syrup and butter? At least now I know that she draws the line of bad eating short of a nonstop orgy of berry-less pancakes.

"So what does Xander drink?"

"He loves juice. I only give him the one hundred percent fruit juice. And usually he has chocolate milk with dinner. And usually with his after school snack. He's got to get his calcium, right?"

"After school snack?"

"He loves nachos, or those little pizza puffs."

Geez, this kid has no chance. Double stacks of pan fried batter swimming in congealed sugar sauce right after waking, deep fried breaded chicken chunks with deep fried potato slivers and corn swimming in cream on the side, all times two at dinner, and interspersed snacks of fried tortilla shards and cheese, and downing glass after glass of liquid calorie concentrate.

"Listen, Kate, you're going to kill Xander by letting him eat all that junk."

"He really will only eat that stuff. I mean, I can't force feed him like when he was a baby, and I don't want him to starve."

"You're his mom, you can choose the stuff he has available to eat. Trust me, he will not starve himself. Look at him, he can probably live for months without eating another bite."

Xander didn't even flinch from his game. He had a quadruple chin looking down at his handheld screen.

"Maybe I will switch him to those 100 calorie snack packs?"

"Changing his diet does not mean only making him eat smaller amounts of the bad stuff. Sure, if I'm choosing between eating a dumpster of garbage versus just a trash can full, I would choose the trash can, but it'd be best not to eat any garbage in the first place. Xander just needs to eat more of the good stuff."

"Dr. Grant, what should I do then?"

"Modest portions, no seconds. Lean meats, try them grilled or baked, not fried. Only water, skim milk or diet drinks for him. No juice, no chocolate milk. Make snacks of raw fresh fruit or vegetables. Make him eat a colorful plate of food, not just browns and darker browns."

"Okay."

"And get him active. Sign him up for some sport, any sport he likes. There are a hundred different sports, and he'll find one he likes. He is way too young to sit in front of the TV all day. "

"How about bowling? He loved it when we went to Brunswick for one of his classmate's birthday party."

Downing pizza and soda while casually flinging an eight pound ball down oiled boards once a week? Then growing up to down pizza and beer while casually flinging a sixteen pound ball down oiled boards once a week in a league? Most bowling leagues are filled with people that look like rolling heart attacks. Everyone looks nine months pregnant with a baby procreated from a combination of beer and having bowling as their only form of exercise. Many can't take the few barely aerobic steps in fast enough sequence for a proper bowling approach so they just grunt their way to the foul line and then rock back and forth to generate a standing swing to generate the meager momentum it takes to get a round, smooth ball to roll down sixty feet of greased wooden boards.

"Umm, I would get him into something with a little more cardio. He needs to get running and jumping at this point."

"Do you hear Dr. Grant, Xander? No more TV and video games all day. And you liked baseball when we played it at grandma's, right? We'll sign you up at the rec center."

I know those are empty words. I've given variations of this speech right into Kate's face countless times, but look at Xander now. He still is a collection of rolls with his candy apple face buried in his GameBoy. She promised to get him more active after every plead, but the only activity I've ever seen him engage in are his thumbs flicking buttons on his video games. He needs to be transported into Super Mario World and spend his days jumping obstacles and dodging Koopa Troopa's. She's such a pushover with Xander. I think he might have eaten her backbone, hickory smoked until fork tender with a side of coleslaw and corn on the cob. Kate was going to graduate to full on enabler in a few years.

"I think that's a great plan, Kate. And if he can get back to a more normal weight soon, he'll probably have fewer problems with those other kids, and he'll just feel better about himself.

You don't want him to be that fat nerd whose life is only computers and fantasy games?"

"Ha ha, I guess not Dr. Grant."

Xander was heading down the narrow road of fat person stereotypes towards his limited place in society. There are many niches a fat kid can fill, and being the nerd is one that is always approving applications. The computer variety seems to be perfect for a lifestyle of extended hours eating junk and sitting on ass. Or he could become an obsessed hobbyist. Gamers, fan boys, Comic-Con conventioneers – many are just groups of fat kids living out more active lives as heroes in a virtual world. They congregate to slather green all over their bodies to become out-of-shape Hulks or squeeze into plastic white armor to become lumpier Stormtroopers. There is also the fat funny guy who can change a laughing-at to a laughing-with (Belushi, Candy, Farley), but Xander's burgeoning introvert makes me think that's not going to be him. Plus, he's never made me laugh with him. The lack of entertaining personality is too bad because he could have a perfect body for radio. If he was an entertaining blabber mouth with personality, he could've spent his days sucking back coffee and donuts seated for hours of drive time in front of a microphone. Television isn't kind to the obese, and is pretty adept at showing contrived

possibilities for fat kids to become: local cops (e.g.
Sipowicz), as part of a comic fat husband/hot wife pair (e.g.
King of Queens), the disgustingly crass male (e.g. Cartman), the
crazily slutty female (e.g. Anna Nicole Smith), Italian mobster
(e.g. Tony Soprano), lovable alcoholic (e.g. Norm Peterson) or
cartoonishly inept all around (e.g. Homer Simpson). The one
positive characterization for the obese is as the fat mascot,
the nice kid everyone likes and keeps around as a second buddy,
but who no one really wants to date - an involuntary eunuch by
means of weight rather than castration. Every attractive
protagonist's best friend needs to be an unattractive, obese
person to accentuate the protagonist's comparative
attractiveness, and that obese person needs an easy going
personality, deep loyalty and a bag of outrageous quips to show
that the protagonist can look past the superficial and befriend
based on more substantive qualities. Xander's outsides are
perfect for that role. But Xander doesn't seem like he's going
to be that great of a friend - one time I asked him for a purple
Skittle and he flat out said no as he poured the rest of the bag
down his throat. My guess is that he's going to end up like
Brian.

Brian was a friend in high school, not a good friend, just
a friend. He was a fat friend. One time we went to the movies

as part of a larger group. I got a large popcorn and a medium Coke (which even back then looked like someone had taken two buckets and filled one with popcorn and one with soda). He got some Skittles. As we were all settling down into our seats, I offered everyone some popcorn. Popcorn and movies? No one can pass that up, especially Brian. He filled his hands with popcorn in between mouthfuls of Skittles. I love purple Skittles, so I asked if I could have one. Brian flat out said no, as he poured the rest of his bag down his throat. Come on, Brian, just one damn Skittle. It would've been just two calories less, just 1/50th of his supply. Yet still no. It was a quick lesson: the fat are greedy for every last calorie. I guess you don't become fat by sharing. And selfishness makes for a bad friend. Brian is now a floor manager in a factory that makes Skittles. And not dating. And really into World of Warcraft and Hentai porn, by rumor.

"So Kate, try to do those things I said, and come back in six months. I want to see a slimmer Xander. I have to see a slimmer Xander."

"I sure will try, Dr. Grant."

Xander finally lifts his head. "Dr. Grant, do you want to play the next game?" as he offers up the console to me.

Kate snatches the GameBoy away. "No, Xander, we're done now. Maybe next time. We have to go to the dentist right now."

"Next time for sure, little buddy. What were you playing?"

"Super Mario. Ha, eating mushrooms makes you so big and I made him eat a lot."

SIX MONTHS FATTER

I walk into the room and it smells great. Smells like
fries. McDonald's fries. Mmm. There's just something about
putting potato in hot grease that makes for good perfume. The
aroma is bad for Xander, though. He's digging into a bag of
McDonald's. He looks bigger. I look down at the vitals in
today's chart and Xander has gained another twenty pounds in six
months.

"Kate, what happened?"

"We tried, Dr. Grant, we really did."

"Did you cut down on his juice and soda?" It was a
rhetorical question at this point as Xander was sucking back on
a super-sized Coke in the examining room.

"He threw such a fit when I tried to take his juice away."

"How about his portions?"

I don't know why I was even asking these questions out loud. This kid was halfway done with a full quarter pounder value meal.

"He complained he was so hungry all of the time when we tried. I don't want to starve my child."

The pangs of hunger can be a friend. An inherent, relatively unpleasant signal that the fuel tank is getting low can be a good warning system to have. The biologic incentive of feeling satiety and quelling those pangs seems like it was a logical Darwinian progression to ensure maintaining the drive of food pursuit. Why risk life and limb and invest all the time to spear a wild boar if eating didn't make you feel better? But nowadays, the pangs of hunger are mostly enemy. The hunt is now ripping open a cellophane wrapper. Hunger is not a signal to eat for survival any longer; it is just a signal to most people that it's time for another two thousand calorie bolus to maintain this oversized fat suit. Yet, hunger is still mistaken for impending death. "Oh my god, I am starving! I better eat something before I die!" said the person looking like he just recently consumed the sum of all the calories needed to be stored in a fallout shelter for a family of four to survive a year underground. I have yet to see a three hundred pounder starve to death. A kid eats a bit less during dinner? Parents freak out and force him to clean his plate before getting any dessert. A kid skips a meal? Better rush him to the doctor and demand a full evaluation for some mystery disease. So parents keep the feedbag on their little porkers to stave off those dangerous hunger pangs. Today, death is more common from too much food rather than too little.

"Did you get him into some cardio activities? Any sports?"

"We tried baseball and soccer. He didn't like it, and the coach was such a mean old guy we had to quit. We have taken him mini-golfing a couple times, though, and he loves that. It's better than nothing, right?"

Better than nothing? It's the same as nothing. I imagine Xander haphazardly knocking his golf ball around with putter in one hand while nursing an ice cream cone in the other. There would be chocolate and vanilla melt around his lips, on his fingers and palms, on the putter grip, on the neon blue ball, and dripping onto the artificial turf. He bends over to grab his ball from the hole and his pants split with a shrill staccato of popping stitches releasing painful tension. People start laughing at him. Xander starts crying. The heaving of his sobs makes his ice cream scoop fall from the cone to the fuzzy plastic green. More crying. Kate runs over and fishes a Snickers from her purse, stuffing it into Xander's hands to try to quell the scene. He starts shrieking about his ice cream, stomping at the ground and sending ripples down his abdominal rolls. Everyone stops their own ice cream eating and putt-putting to stare, shaking their heads at Xander, which also causes their own massive bellies to ripple from side to side. Rain starts falling and the ice cream melt flows down towards the hole, circling away as if into a drain.

"You know, Kate, there are summer camps dedicated to overweight kids. Maybe that's what he needs, a separation from his usual routines."

"We tried something like that, but on the second day of fat camp, Xander fell down playing kickball and hit his head, so we had to pull him out of the program."

"Okay."

"I mean, he burst his forehead open! What kind of supervision is that? Xander has a real high pain tolerance so when I heard he was crying, I knew he was really hurt. I had to force them to rush Xander to the Emergency Room. When I met him there, I literally could see his skull through his cut!"

"Well, I can't imagine..."

"Then the ER doc there tries to say he can close it with some glue. No way! Not for my baby's face! I had to force the doc there to call in a plastic surgeon to repair the gushing cut. Xander had to be put under for the repair, but look at his face, it was worth it."

I peered over at Xander's forehead and saw a half centimeter line of lighter skin. This was the life threatening gash? There was no way it was more than just a scrape. Kate implying severity based on Xander's crying despite his pain tolerance was ridiculous. Every parent says their kid has a high pain tolerance, so much so that the claim has no meaning. No parent is going to admit that their kid is a babied wimp created from their constant helicoptering and persistent positive feedback from exaggerated overjoyed reactions over trivial happenings. In reality, most kids like Xander will cry murder even if a ladybug flutters onto their arm. And calling in a plastic surgeon for that little nick? A surgeon trained to reconstruct massive deformity being demanded by some mom to put a suture into a fleck of a laceration? This wound did not heal this well because of the gifted hands of the plastic surgeon; it would've healed just like it did even if Xander sealed it shut himself with a thumb of mud. Why not demand that the Pope come and irrigate it with fresh holy water before closure? Then maybe get Jesus to float down and seal the cut with his healing finger? It's no wonder Xander gets all his demands filled to excess.

"Kids get minor scrapes when they are active, it's entirely normal and impossible to always prevent. Xander needs to get active, regardless of those minor risks. And most cuts and bruises will heal just fine and are not that big of a deal."

"Well, next time, we're going to have to find a better supervised program."

"A small cut is not that high of a price to pay if it means Xander is getting healthier."

"I guess."

"Regardless Kate, you've really done nothing we talked about and it shows. Xander is up another twenty pounds."

"We'll keep trying, but it's tough."

"You're his mom, you need to do this for him. I shouldn't be caring about this more than you."

"I know, I know." Kate sighed.

Xander finished his lunch, and with a burp, tossed the McDonald's bag into the trash. Next stop: World of warcraft and Hentai porn. This kid has got no chance. No fucking chance.

FAT BULLY

About once a month, I do a free sports physical clinic at a
local grade school. It's a good way to provide some physicals
for kids that otherwise wouldn't get one. And occasionally, I
will see some minor urgent care stuff - strains, runny noses,
rashes and such.

On one visit to Jane Adams Elementary, as my mind started
getting numb from the repetition of normal pediatric physicals,
Xander was escorted into the exam room. A burly teacher had a
tight grip on Xander's right upper arm. Xander had a cut on his
left hand and a zig-zagged scratch on the center of his forehead
a la Harry Potter. He was almost as wide as he was tall.

"Hey Xander, long time no see, how's it going buddy?"

The teacher that was escorting him just shook his head.
"Not too good, he was beating up a kid again."

Makes sense. Xander's been getting called "Lardass" and
"Triple ex-el-Xander" for a few years now, and that's a perfect
recipe to get bitter and mean. And by the looks of him, he was
just eating more junk to cope. But he must've also figured out
that at this age, his body used that excess fuel to grow wider
and taller at a quicker rate than his peers. Like how the grass
where the neighborhood dogs squat their crap grows lushest. He
became the biggest kid in class. Suddenly, he found another,
more satisfying way to feel better: beating on kids. I wish I
could've been there when one kid too many called Xander "Fat-
fuck", and Xander reared back and connected with the kid's face,
sending the kid flying. Like a semi-truck hitting a Prius. And
a lightbulb going off that mass was strength, at least at this
pre-pubertal age.

"Let's take a look at him."

Xander just had some superficial scratches and minor soft
tissue swelling. More so on his knuckles. That kid he was
beating on must have got lit up.

"Anything hurt, Xander?"

"No, not really, Dr. Grant."

I took his hand and started feeling around. "Not here, or
here?"

"No, not really."

Then this teacher chimed in, "Are you sure nothing's broken? Because my cousin got in a fight once and he broke his hand. Never healed right because the doc missed it."

I'm going to ignore this guy. What did he think I was doing, not making sure it wasn't broken? If so, the unsolicited consult from the peanut gallery will surely crack the case. I also once had a cousin that got wasted on Jim Beam and punched a clown at a circus, so maybe Xander is drunk right now? Everyone likes to play armchair doctor, thinking their secondhand medical knowledge is fact, but most need to just sit quiet in that armchair and realize they are uninformed. This is the type of guy that would Google some symptoms and read some website for an hour and then fight a doctor's reasoned diagnosis with his own dim brainstorm by claiming he had done his research -- that is not research. Research is done by multiply degreed scientists that devote their lives to advancing knowledge meticulously; research is done by committees of scientists reviewing hundreds of studies on their scientific robustness to come to an evidence based conclusion; research is done by physicians, who were trained for over a decade to have a skeptical eye, then reviewing committee conclusions and medical journals for skepticism-quashing robustness to reach a threshold to apply evidence based recommendations to clinical practice. Scrolling a random blog for an hour is not research. Don't read a placemat then try to convince me that it's *The New England Journal of Medicine*. Don't solve the kiddy word jumble on the placemat then claim to have cracked some far reaching scientific mystery. Knowing someone who had something at sometime for some reason is not a basis for diagnosis.

"Xander's all right, he's good to go."

The teacher grabbed Xander's arm, leaned closer to him and got serious. "Xander, this is your third fight this month. You're going to be suspended for sure. And why are you beating on little Sam, he's half your size."

Kids should only tremble in fear of Xander if they were shipwrecked on a food-less island and were covered in butter, not here in school where there are dozens of vending machines to pump out seemingly unlimited amounts of Doritos and Snickers for Xander to feed his sour moods. But food must've not been enough to fill all of Xander's holes. "What did little Sam do to deserve such a beating?"

The teacher gave Xander's arm a squeeze. "Tell him."

Xander just shrugged.

"Tell Dr. Grant that you didn't like Sam's cardigan with Snoopy and Woodstock on it, and how you beat him down so you could rip it off him."

Fat people are supposed to be jolly. Santa is Jolly Ol'
Saint Nick. The Kool-Aid Man bursts through brick walls and
offers cool refreshment with a bellowing chuckle. Imagine a
stereotypical cheery grandmother baking cookies; she is, in the
least, generously overweight. Are fat people all just gentle
souls whose become sullied by society's harsh mocking? But then
there's Jabba the Hut. Or Rush Limbaugh. Or Tony Soprano.
Turns out, jerks come in all sizes. The jerk gene does not
discriminate. Fat people always spout that they want to one day
have their outsides be as beautiful as their insides, as if
being overweight automatically qualifies a person as being
internally good with a dyssynchrony of physique and personality.
It is easy to hide personality failings behind the theoretical
effects of the perceived slights of others onto the voluntary
elections of outward appearance, but the fact is that no one
wants to admit that their outsides may be just as bloated and
disfigured as their insides. Obesity could just as easily be a
symptom of self-absorption, selfishness and stinginess. Hell,
neither Xander nor Brian would share even one damn purple
Skittle with me.

Bullying is about power, and most, no matter their size,
will happily take power given its therapeutic effects on some
internal ill. In particular, grade school bullies are usually

the fat kid that just uses his weight advantage to pound kids.
The bully just started out eating too much, got fat, got called
fatty-fat-fat, then got bitter, ate more to feel better, got
even fatter, then realized it's easy to overpower kids that
weigh half your size. And kids will respect someone that can
beat up other kids. I bet Xander is real popular now. Suddenly
kids become impressed rather than disgusted when Xander eats
four bologna sandwiches for lunch. Xander now gets picked
first for recess football because he can carry would-be tacklers
into the end zone as if they were kids hanging on the sides of a
train headed to Darjeeling. And with all that positive
feedback, now Xander finds it hilarious pounding on a kid who
loves *Peanuts*.

"Is the kid Xander beat up coming to clinic?"

The teacher shook his head. "We sent him to the hospital.
Xander sat on his face for a while and some kids said Sam might
have stopped breathing for a while."

I almost laughed aloud. A kid almost killed by smothering
fat rolls. Xander sent to death row for murder in the first by
a fat-ass ass. The kid should've tried to fight Xander by
continually shuffling away just out of reach; Xander would've no
doubt died of a heart attack if he chased the kid more than half
a block. Xander looked like he could die of a heart attack just

from walking to a soda machine. He was a walking heart attack in grade school.

It is too bad that grade school bully weight will eventually became a disadvantage. Puberty will hit and it will turn out that fat weight is very different from muscle weight. When other kids hit puberty, they will gain muscle mass because their intake is balanced enough to create good mass rather than having to store bad mass. Xander's state of intake will make him a super-sized storage facility for bad mass. I bet puberty for Xander will mean acne, nocturnal emissions and non-stop fast food. Topical benzoyl peroxide will tame the acne, masturbation will offer release from the emissions, but his weight will never meet the salve of diet and exercise. It will become the festering sore that only gets worse. I bet puberty for little Sam will be developing a Napoleon complex and starting to lift weights with an angry passion, then quelling his internal ills by beating on fat kids when he develops into a fire hydrant of a linebacker. Xander's just getting his time in the bully sun before it's too late.

The teacher started pulling Xander out of the room.

"Say hi to your mom for me, Xander."

"Okay, Dr. Grant."

JUNIOR

When Xander rolled in for his seventh grade physical, it was
apparent he was dedicated to going the route of bigger being
better. For medical purposes, kids' weights are measured in
kilograms; Xander was eighty kilograms when he should've been
eighty pounds. And now he was sporting Buddy Holly glasses.
And going out in public in dirty sweatpants and a T-shirt with a
smiling whale cartoon on the front set under the words "Whales
are fun!".

Seventh grade is the start of some heightened social
awareness - puberty starts for most, the opposite sex become
noticed, and being cool stops being about baseball cards and
Barbies. Seeing Xander in sweats and a marine wildlife tee as a
seventh grader was concerning.

"Hey Kate, how's Xander doing?"

"He's doing real well."

Xander had his head buried in a book entitled "Marine Biology".

"What activities is he doing now?"

"He's really taken to swimming. He's goes all the time at the club."

It looks like he needs to go more. Whatever calories he's burning by swimming is just mist evaporating off an ocean of eating, for sure. Fat does float, though. I imagine him floating on his back in the shallow end peeling into a Snickers bar, looking like an otter cracking into a clam.

"How's he doing at school?"

"Really great. Ever since he watched something on whales on National Geographic, all he talks about is wanting to be a marine biologist. I mean, his bedroom is wall to wall pictures of turtles, whales, manatees, sharks…"

Kate went on for another few minutes naming more sea wildlife. Curious that she thinks I don't get it that Xander is now obsessed with marine biology, and that the only way to convince me is by listing animals that live in or near oceans. It's always good to have interests but becoming this obsessed, this early, turns Xander from the "fat kid" to the "weird fat kid into whales". Kids are just going to call him a whale. It is really concerning that either Xander doesn't see the obvious fodder or that he doesn't care.

"...and sea anemomes. It's really given him motivation to do well in school. I even brought his report card to show you."

Kate fished around in her Dior purse for a while. She had on matching Gucci shoes and a revealing Gucci tunic. I didn't know Gucci made anything besides purses.

"I can't find it here. Oh, Xander do you have it? Show Dr. Grant your report card, Xander."

Xander reached into his book and fished out a slip of paper, holding it out for me without lifting his head from his book. I took the report card. All A's, and one D. In gym.

"What happened in gym, little buddy."

"Gym is stupid."

"Why is it stupid?"

"Because it is."

Preteens are usually jerkfaces to any adult, especially to their doctor, but this smelled different. It smelled familiar.

I knew a kid named Michael Ferry who was in most of my gifted classes in junior high - we called him "Fat Ferry". He was however a surprisingly popular kid for being a five-four, two hundred thirty pound scumbag. Scumbag in the sense that he wore the same zebra striped pants everyday with an array of T-

shirts that seemed to be more sweat and grease than cotton. He
was undoubtedly popular from the fact that he dabbled in smoking
and selling weed.

Every fall, every seventh and eighth grader would have to
run the mile for a grade in gym. There would be some training
runs for a week or so to gear us up for the final run, and the
hope was that the final run would be a personal best. Better
times meant better grades, and slacking was punished with a redo
of the mile, so there was good motivation to put in at least
some effort. Michael was the kid that pitted out his T-shirt
just walking to the starting line and ran the training miles in
over thirty minutes. Most of the days he was late to our next
period's math class because he couldn't finish the one mile in
the allotted gym class time. And he usually spent the hour of
advanced algebra breathing heavy and sweating through his tee,
with a zombie-like blank stare and gaping mouth. But whatever,
it was no big deal to most of the other kids because it was not
a surprise, and Michael didn't get ripped with ridicule, mainly
due to the fact that half the gym class was impressed with a
twelve year old kid that could get weed.

Well, that ended. Michael shit his shorts during the final
mile run.

I remember almost everyone was finishing up their last four hundred meters, and Michael was still working his way to the halfway point, so there were plenty of people still lapping him around the track. Then some commotion.

"Shit! It's shit!"

"What the fuck, he shit!"

Everyone scattered and halted their running. Michael just collapsed onto the grass.

Word was that Michael threw it into the infield grass. That stress shit must've been in his shorts for at least a little while before he got the nerve to reach into his shorts and try to toss the evidence into the grass. Hey, it's just goose shit, or someone must've walked their dog here sometime. A gallant try to rid the proof of his acutely increased parasympathetic tone, but that's when he got caught. He might have been better off keeping it in his pants, but then again, he still had more than half a mile to run and a shorts-full of the sloppy slurry from his sweat, shit and friction would've been intolerable. It was the epitome of a no win situation – the mind hazy from lack of oxygen, the body weak from maximal exertion, and fresh shit in the tightie used-to-be whities. He got sent to the nurse, and then sent home.

Michael was not too popular after that. Didn't matter how much weed he smoked or sold, he became the kid that shit his pants. Someone also started a rumor a week later that he pissed his pants during a Social Studies exam. Since it was proven he was able to become totally incontinent of stool, it was only a small leap to take to peg him as incontinent of urine too. And in light of him recently shitting his shorts, he had no credibility in denying any excrement related stories, even though I have yet to find anyone that actually saw his piss on pants. He did eventually amp up his drug use to coke. He got arrested in high school for gun possession and went into the juvenile justice system. Last I heard was that Michael is locked up in the state penitentiary serving ten to twenty for dealing heroin.

The slight bit of good news here was that only drug Xander looked to be on was cheeseburgers.

"Xander, did you run the mile in gym?"

"Last week I did."

"Did you poop your pants?"

"What? No."

From his tone I could tell he really hadn't. I guess Xander is just a shitless Fat Ferry. He hates gym because he just sucks at gym.

"You know Xander, marine biologists need to be in good shape to get down to the wildlife they want to study. Swimming, climbing ocean shorelines, exploring deep waters – you need to be fit in order to do all that. And gym class is a great opportunity to get some exercise every day to start getting healthy for a career in marine biology."

I thought that little pep talk was pretty good for just having made all of it up in streaming thought. Kate perked up. "That's so true, honey, and you want to be a good marine biologist, right?"

Xander just nodded.

"Jacque Cousteau was a fit guy, and he was one of the most famous marine biologists ever." Another stroke of inspiration. Who knows if that's even true, but I always picture Captain Nemo from the movie "20,000 Leagues Under the Sea" when I think of Jacque and that captain was a fit enough guy to beat on a giant squid and survive an angry tentacle grasp.

Xander finally looked up from his book. "I will try harder in gym."

That's nice. It's a bunch of crap, but it's still nice. The world could use another Jacque Cousteau. Even an overweight one. But the amount of time and effort it would take for Xander to even get back to average fitness was massive, certainly

dwarfing the medicine droppers of help thirty minutes of half-
hearted gym class activity would ever add. It's a vicious

circle for fat kids in gym: so big they can't compete with the

other kids, so they don't put in as much effort as the other

kids, so they become even less competitive, then they get tossed

to the sidelines, then they put in even less effort, so that

eventually gym becomes thirty minutes of standing against padded

walls on hardwood. Not enough activity to even burn off a can

of soda. And having a teacher whose primary credentials are

being able to wear shorts and inflate various balls doesn't help

with instilling motivation. Neither is the seeping sentiment

that gym is extraneous – it's always the first to meet the axe

with any significant district budget cuts. Gym was not going to

crack Xander's case.

   Obviously, Xander's physical exam was not good. Belly skin

full of stretch marks. His midsection looked like pulled peach

play-doh. The back of his neck had dark velvety skin --

acanthosis nigicans – a sign of insulin resistance, a stop on

the road to diabetes. Most of his teeth were more fillings than

native tooth, and new festering cavities gave his exhalations a

sour punch. He sounded like he was out of breath from just

hopping on and off the exam table. He was marinating in a thin

layer of sweat that made him feel clammy all over, and look

greasy as if he'd been manning the fry station and absorbing the oil splatter at McDonald's all day. He smelled subtly of old world cheese.

"Well, Kate, I'm not going to say anything new…"

Sighing, "Yeah, we know, Xander has to lose weight."

"And I'm going to send Xander for some blood work today: fasting blood sugar, lipid panel, insulin and liver enzymes. And thyroid function, too."

Kate brightened a bit. "You think that could be it? Hypothyroidism?"

The dream is that all Xander needs is a pill once a day to fix all of his ills. Just like most parents, she is holding on to hope that her child's abnormality is due to some disease outside of her or the child's control. It's much better than acknowledging that he's just fat because he's fat. How convenient would it be to shift personal responsibility to some tangible condition beyond a person's control? The next stop will be to say Xander has an addiction to food, that he has the "disease" of addiction, to compare him to a hypothetical heroin addict that has to use a little bit of heroin three times a day to get nutrients. Total crap. A person can get all their needed nutrients eating flavorless greens and meats if they wanted to do so. I have yet to meet the obese person claiming a

food addiction that got fat eating dry salad and boiled skinless
chicken. Xander is not addicted to food. He just enjoys the
feeling of food that tastes good to him, just like everybody
else, but he has chosen to forgo common sense and eat
ridiculously high amounts of processed and instant gratification
calorie dense foods because they taste the best to him and are
more easily consumed, consequences be damned. He made a series
of poor decisions that morphed into a bad habit consisting of
nothing but continued poor food decisions. Obviously habits can
be hard to break, but habits are just habits and are not
ingrained into his DNA like his sex, so they can be eliminated
with a convicted decision to modify behavior. If Kate was
really serious about helping to rid his problem with food, she
could just eliminate the overvalued highs that Xander has placed
on tastiness. If certain foods cause problems, make the
decision to eliminate them. Keep them out of the house. Make
it harder to find those foods. Don't let him have a taste, then
decide to limit the problem food; the decision for control has
to be made beforehand. Just have him eat home prepared meals
only. Just have him eat raw vegetables and legumes every meal -
not as delicious as bacon cheeseburgers, but it will stave off
overeating, provide daily nutrients, and begin the journey of
weight loss. But that would mean difficult sacrifice with only

an abstract promise of a future healthier life - too much work for an unseen reward. So he will never give up his diet of deep fried fats. Kate would rather look for medical conditions that could be blamed for his weight and continue to allow him to wallow in his woe-is-me obesity.

This hope for a medical disease diagnosis is the same as when Xander started doing a bit worse in school earlier this year. Kate cried it was ADHD. Again, total crap. No kid develops ADHD for the first time at Xander's current age. Furthermore, though some kids really do have the disorder, nowadays, it's a reason attributed by any parent for their kid with poor school performance. It's easier to say their kid has a disorder that prevents focus, rather than admit the kid is just not that smart. By simple normal distribution curve, more kids are going to be average to below-average than above-average; not everyone is going to crack physics and organic chemistry, most are going to do well to balance their checkbooks and read checkout line magazines. But ADHD can be treated with a pill, so parents would rather have their kid labeled with a condition that can be ameliorated with medicine than be labeled as just being average. The ideal diagnoses for a dumb, fat kid for most parents would be ADHD and hypothyroidism, where a couple pills once a day would transform mind and body from Shrek to Captain America. There is no pill that will ever cancel out Xander eating as much crap as he wants.

"No, I don't think that hypothyroidism is that likely, but I think these labs are worth checking at this point."

"Ooh, let's hope that's what it is."

"Kate, most of these labs are to see if he's got some other medical problems related to his obesity, not really to look for a reason for his obesity. We know he consumes too many calories and lives a sedentary lifestyle – that's going to be the real reason."

Xander hadn't looked up from his book the whole time we were talking, but now his head shot up to meet his mom's face, "Can you guys please shut up? I'll try harder in gym, okay?"

Kate just stared at him. They stared at each other for a while. I stared at them. I guess his mom's unbridled glee at the prospect of him having some endocrine disorder was too much even for his teenage apathetic disposition. Time for me to end this visit.

"Okay, so, I'll have the nurse come in and get you those lab requisition forms."

Xander returned to his book while Kate continued staring. I left the room fast and quiet. Just as if he was a jar of

mayonnaise left out in the midday sun, this fatty was starting
to sour.

.

FAT FROSH?

"What the hell happened to you, Xander?"

For his freshman physical, I expected to see a pizza faced blob with a curtain of greasy hair 360 degrees from scalp to shoulders in an attempt to cover up the facial train wreck, and clothes baggy and black to camouflage his girth. Adding hormones to a pot of fat is usually never pretty. Instead, Xander was tall and only mildly overweight, and with a more muscular frame. His hair was short and tousled in place with gel. And he was in jeans and a Matt Forte jersey. He looked like a fitter Chicago-bred Yogi Bear.

"I cut out soda and Gatorade, and I joined the football team. Those two-a-days were brutal."

Kate was smiling ear-to-ear. She was looking at Xander as if gazing upon him for the first time after he emerged from a 15 hour labor. "Albert played football in college, so Xander

thought he'd give it a try, and he's doing great."

   She was glowing. Her hair was up in a tight bun, she had on

rimless glasses, a cashmere turtleneck, wool skirt and knee-high

leather boots. She looked like the sexy librarian that could

draw men to rehearse small talk on the Dewey Decimal System.

Too bad I sent her out of the room. Xander was fourteen; he

doesn't need his mommy for his physicals anymore. There are

going to questions that most teens will never answer honestly in

front of their parents. Plus, no teenage boy wants his mom to

catch a glimpse of his weiner during the hernia check.

   I wish I could take some credit for Xander's lifestyle

change and weight loss, but the truth is that all my warning and

lecturing and pleading with Kate and Albert, and repeating the

same diction to Xander himself, probably penetrated like bullets

into Wonder Woman's bracelets. No one really gives a shit what

their doctor says; words from a lab-coated nerd are not

motivation to do anything. The motivation to lose weight is

usually comes from a small catalog of possibilities: getting

sick of shame and ridicule, realizing life is getting shittier

and shorter because of fat, or getting a taste of something

better than food. Sometimes that tipping point comes from being

led off an amusement park ride in front of a winding line of snickering, impatient people because even with the efforts of multiple attendants, the safety belt just couldn't get around. Or keeling over with crushing chest pain while walking to work during the morning rush, and because it takes multiple attempts by two paramedics and three passerbyers to get loaded into the ambulance, and because time is cardiac muscle, a minor heart attack gets delayed into a major one and produces lengthened time for in-hospital contemplation. Xander changed because he got a taste of something better than food. Xander got a taste of being a jock, being part of a team, and didn't mind passing on a few cheeseburgers to have more peeps, parties and panties roll his way.

"Alright Xander, I'm going to start by asking you a few questions I ask all teenagers."

"Okay."

"Ever use alcohol?"

"Nope."

"Tobacco?"

"Never."

"Drugs?"

"Nope."

"Any of your friends use drugs?"

"Unless you count Xbox as a drug."

"How about supplements?"

"No, I don't think taking some weird herb can actually make you better at sports."

"Steroids?"

"C'mon, Dr. Grant, that's just stupid. And I'm not even close to being that ripped. I look barely muscled, much less over-muscled. And who wants a pizza for a back and a pair of honey roasted peanuts for testes?"

"Hey, I have to ask or I wouldn't be doing my job, right?" Xander smiled with a shrug. "Have you ever been sexually active?"

"Yes."

Whoa. Looks like Xander's weight loss really opened a lot of doors for him. He was a pretty good looking kid with his extra weight gone. Seems like that is how most overweight people are: attractive people hiding underneath layers and layers of adipose. Watch the mommy weight loss episodes of *Oprah*, or read the weight loss human interest stories in *People*, or turn in for the entire arc of *The Biggest Loser* - usually the people that have to lose over fifty percent of their body weight in order to return to average turn out to be good looking people. Of course it helps that those publicized images tend to have good lighting and makeup and editors, a tight selection

process, access to photoshop and a horrible "before" comparison
image, but regardless, these once obese people could easily be a
cast for a potential GAP ad. It seems like Xander was living
the life of an attractive person now.

"How many partners for you, Xander?"

"Forty. Forty-seven if you count prostitutes."

"What?"

"Ha, ha, gotcha doc. I've never been sexually active. Did
you see what I looked like before? Not many girls want to get
boned by a beanbag chair with a little smokie sticking out of
it. Plus, I don't think mom would be cool with becoming a
grandmother right now."

Xander has gotten hilarious. A new physique, a new
personality - Xander was on his way to becoming a heartwarming
story. Though under the mesh of his jersey, I could see he was
wearing a T-shirt with an Emperor penguin on it. It was even
more impressive that he still held true to his geeky interior
while changing his exterior. He was still holding onto the
remnants of the old Xander, but he played football now, so who
cares? A fat kid with a marine animal shirt is a flaming nerd,
but an athlete with a penguin on his shirt is cool because he's
a brainiac meathead - a guy that could wear something other than
popped Lacoste polos and loose Buffalos, and by seemingly not

caring what other kids think, he was actually making them think sea mammalian tees were approaching kitschy cool. His confidence could make him a trendsetter in his small teenaged world.

"Well if you ever decide to become sexually active, you know you can always come here to talk about it. Anything you say will be confidential. By law, your mom will not hear about anything from me."

I never thought I would ever need to give Xander a sex talk. Morbid obesity is the ultimate birth control. Sure, a few obese girls and boys sometimes get opportunity to act really slutty to even out the playing field, but morbidly obese people have such a limited selection of potential suitors, that natural selection usually takes care of their teenage pregnancy rates. But, this new Xander is now high risk. Improving his chances to get his pig-into-a-blanket was obviously part of his drive to lose weight, so in that end, Xander, mission accomplished.

"That's good to know, Dr. Grant. What if I said all I fantasize about is that while I'm boning some chick, I slowly put a pillow over her face so she's trashing for breath when I climax?"

Holy shit. "Well, uh, in that instance...hmmm..."

"C'mon Dr. G, I'm joking. Oh man, you should have seen the look on your face."

This kid is my kind of kid, now. I looked down at his vitals in the chart: good heart rate, good blood pressure, weight trending down towards a normal BMI. Nice. His physical exam was largely normal, save for a few fading stretch marks around his abdominal flanks. He had markedly better strength and flexibility than I remembered from his physical last year. He could do a duck walk across the exam room without breaking a sweat. He looked well-built for football. I guess that makes sense: how could he not have had some baseline muscle mass after having had enough fat draped on him as to basically be in a constant state of weightlifting?

"Xander, I have to tell you, this new you is really, really great. You've lost weight, gained muscle mass, you seem happy and look healthier - just fantastic, little buddy."

Xander just smiled. "Thanks, Dr. Grant."

"What has your diet been like recently?"

"Well, like I told you before, I cut out all drinks except for water or diet soda..."

"Awesome."

"...but I guess my diet is still pretty typical teenager - still some junk. Like the whole team goes to grab pizza and

burgers after almost every practice and game, and you know how
it goes, eating a lot is a male pride thing."

"Well, just be careful with that, because your metabolism
is the best it's ever going to be right now, so you can eat
total garbage at this age and your body will just burn it.
But, if you keep with the bad eating habits, as your metabolism
slows down as you get older, your body is not going to be able
to burn it all and you will put on weight. You are not going to
be doing two-a-days when you're fifty."

"God, I hope I don't still have to do those then."

"I am not saying you can't eat some junk, but do it in
moderation, and try eating some more fruits and veggies."

"Alright, doc, I will try my best. Junk tastes so good,
though."

"Yeah, I know. But the key words here are "in moderation".
A life without some junk would not be too enjoyable. Sometimes,
nothing is better than a good bacon cheeseburger."

"Or an Italian beef with giardiniera."

"Or a deep dish Lou's pizza." Imagining that cheesy deep
dish pie was making my mouth water. I suddenly got depressed
thinking about the sack lunch I packed today of turkey and swiss
on whole wheat with a side of sliced apples. "Anyway Xander,

you're going great, just keep it up, and try to do a bit better on your food choices."

"Will do. And no more 'tutes, eh?"

"What?"

"Prosti-tutes. I should cut down on handies from them too, right?"

This kid was downright hilarious. As he left the exam room, my pen bounced from line to line in his chart and every other word seemed to be "good" or "improved". His change happened in such a relative blink, to the point of puzzlement that it did not happen sooner. With so much abject failure in the practice of medicine, even a glimmer of possible success makes for rainbows and bunnies. Today's Xander is what makes the slog through the hellhole of clownish patients worthwhile. I saw him now going on morning runs with his wife, hiking through the Grand Canyon, chasing kids across greenery, chasing grandkids across greenery, and spryly hopping into a hover car. Before today, it seemed I wanted that long life for him more than he did. Long live this new Xander.

WATERMELON TOOTHPICK

Every Fourth of July, the country club holds a barbeque for
all the members and their families. It is always a great
spread, great fireworks, and a good time. I haven't been in
attendance for a while, but somehow all my other plans fell
through this summer holiday, so I went. Albert, Kate and Xander
were there as usual.

"Dr. Grant! Great to see you!" Kate ran over from the
buffet line and gave me a hug.

Albert and Xander were just finishing loading their plates,
and they headed over towards me, faces lighting up and waving.
Xander was balancing two plates heaped with pulled pork and ribs
peeking out under coleslaw, corn-on-the-cob and beans. He was

waddling. It looked like every step was a battle of leg and
ground, and the jackhammer shocks of his foot strikes unable to
be dissipated by the matted grass seemed to be sending
reverberations of pain back up to his already damaged joints.

I hadn't seen Xander in a few years. He was old enough now
to be able to decide to ignore the recommendation to see his
doctor once a year, and certainly he's old enough to not need a
pediatrician. Seeing him heavier and hobbling was surprising,
considering the last time I saw him, he was an emerging jock and
turning his way down a healthier path. Usually high school
football players add the pounds gradually after they stop
playing, trading muscle for fat by continuing to eat and drink
as if they were still in practices every day and with a
teenager's metabolism. Xander did have an elastic brace on his
right knee. It was probably the result of an old football
injury. Probably the reason he had to stop football. Probably
the reason he was able to put on so many pounds so quickly.
Though probably not that serious of an injury because the brace
he was wearing was only adding a whisker of additional support
in relation to the body mass his knee was supporting on a step
by step basis. That injury had to have happened years ago in
high school, so why still with the ineffectual brace? Maybe for
placebo effect? More likely for show to provide an excuse and

point of sympathy for being sedentary. The injury was moot. It was his obscene body habitus that was making him gimpy now.

Imagine supporting a marshmallow on a couple toothpicks - easy. Now try balancing an apple, then a cantaloupe, then a watermelon on those same two toothpicks. Joints and cartilage and bursas are amazing feats of anatomic engineering, but they are missing a weight limit sign, so people assume the sky is the limit. Pain starts from weighted bone grinding away all the cushioning in between bones, in the way of mortar and pestle, and pain pathways become exposed and persistently agitated because the weights of five average people are abusing a single joint. With every step, his joints scream out in throes of spikes underneath fingernails torture. Pain prevents exercise. Pain prevents even walking. Pain is eased with barbeque. More pain is eased with more barbeque. The apple becomes a cantaloupe becomes a watermelon. Then snapped toothpicks. This is a twenty-eight year old guy looking like he's going to need a Rascal in a couple months. Xander had already started to wear out his joints before reaching middle age. But, I guess the way he's going, this could be his middle age.

"Hey Dr. Grant, great to see you. You should really try some of this pork." Xander had enough pork on his plate to re-form an entire pig. Lunch time with the obese. Very rarely have I seen in person someone obese put down a full extra-large sausage and pepperoni pizza or four Big Mac meals in one sitting. Usually the amount of food I observe being consumed is at the upper limits of a reasonable portion - of course that portion already having been arbitrarily bloated by mass consumer gluttony - but still, all I have ever seen one person put down live is a super-sized value meal plus a few dessert extras like a sundae and an individual apple pie. Most consume the additional calories by in-taking constantly throughout the day or with more substantial amounts in solitude. Even gluttons realize outsized gluttony in public will elicit circus side show stares, so they attempt to avoid the murmurs by making their gluttony a private sin. Not Xander anymore. Xander's plate surpasses the threshold of a reasonable portion, easily. He had gotten to the stage where if anyone watched him eat any meal, they would understand how he was able to achieve and maintain all his adipose.

"I sure will, Xander, that looks real good. Hi Albert, long time no see."

"It has been a while for sure, good to see you." As Albert extended his hand for a shake, his cell phone started ringing. The ringtone was the Notre Dame fight song. He unlatched the phone from his belt and looked down at the caller ID. "Ooh, sorry, I have to take this." Albert excused himself and took the call. Meanwhile, Xander was already chewing away, in between heaving breaths. Breathing seemed to be a nuisance to his eating. He had let his hair grow to shoulder length, and it looked like his mop had never met comb. He looked like a lazy roadie. He also looked seven months pregnant. All his overeating and fat storage in the past had made it too easy for him to pack the weight back. All those extra fat cells created from years of massive calories, then being continually filled to the maximum had set him up for effortless obesity for life. Even with those cells being emptied through a comparatively brief detour towards fitness in high school, the infrastructure was always in place for a quick refill. How much easier is it to refill pre-existing containers than to get the raw materials to make containers, make new containers, and then fill them?

Kate just frowned. "Xander, slow down, you sound like you're choking on your food."

It didn't sound anything like choking. It sounded more rhythmic, like air escaping from an over-inflated air mattress as grandma tosses and turns to sleep. He was literally out of breath just standing there eating, almost gasping, as if air was just another piece of pork needing to be gorged. It makes sense; try breathing with a fifty pound weight on your chest.

Try breathing after letting your conditioning decline to a point where eating becomes aerobic exercise. Try breathing while your heart and lungs struggle to meet the demands of an ever-expanding body. Even the simple act of breathing becomes exhausting, making for more exhaustive breathing.

"Man, it sure is hot out here," as he wiped away streams of perspiration from his forehead. It was maybe seventy-five degrees with a slight breeze -- very pleasant. I was even wearing a light jacket. Kate was just in a thin formfitting white dress shirt and khakis. Xander was in a pitted-out Shedd Aquarium T-shirt and baggy jeans. This guy has the eat-sweats. He was in a state of gustatory bliss where his body was pumping so much pleasure catecholamines on the inside to the point of needing to pour liquid chlorides from every pore on the outside.

No anti-perspirant was going to contain that onslaught. When downing barbeque becomes a near maximal aerobic activity, the body starts to react as if it were perpetually exercising. Sweat becomes a second skin. Sweat on a beautiful woman is glistening dew; this sweat is juice escaping from a cooking sausage link, the pepperoni pizza oil seeping through a paper bag. And it is perpetual. Sweat collects in countless flaps and crevasses, and marinates the body in salty exudate, so now the fat guy is the clammy, smelly fat guy. Those dark, humid and rarely cleaned fat roll pockets must be feeding bonanzas for all sorts of foul bacteria and fungi. Luckily, I was upwind so all I smelled was the smoke from the grill.

Kate fished a napkin from her purse and blotted Xander's forehead. "Pace yourself, honey, the grill is going to be cooking all day until the fireworks, so take it easy. No need to rush the plates. You're really sweating."

"Okay mom I'll try, but come on, it's the Fourth."

He was right; it was the Fourth of July. And since it was a holiday, it was one of the socially excused days to gorge for most people: New Years Eve filet and crab legs, Easter champagne brunch buffet, Memorial Day barbeque, Fourth of July barbeque, Labor Day barbeque, Thanksgiving turkey with all the fixings, and Christmas ham with all the fixings. And the Super Bowl spread every year. And don't forget all the birthdays of family and friends and the friends of family and friends to be celebrated. And engagements and weddings. And graduations. And getting pregnant and being pregnant and then celebrating having the actual babies. And new jobs, and leaving jobs, and doing something good at your job. And the end of the week and the start of a new week. And vacations. Pretty much at least once a week there is an excuse to spend a day doing nothing else but eat massive quantities of delicious, unhealthy food. An

extra hundred calories a day makes for a gain of about ten
pounds a year; just an extra can of soda, an extra two Oreos, an
extra few bites of pizza that are not burned off each day will
get the average guy to three hundred pounds in about ten years.
But no one overeats by just a handful of M&M's. It's more
likely that it is overeating by a few handfuls of M&M's on top
of each handful of M&M's. Just these occasions to over consume
make for at least a thousand extra calories, and that is in
addition to the every day, non-special occasion surplus
consumption of calories, so a few thousand extra calories a week
can easily become the norm. It is as if consumption was assumed
to be a God given right. As if God had commanded every warm-
blooded human to go forth and multiply their fat cells in
perpetuity. And any effort to challenge that entitlement is met
with mind-boggling resistance, as if trying to advise healthy
diet and exercise is an intrusion into some Constitutional
freedom. It's no wonder most of the men here at the club were
wearing tent-sized Lacoste polos with most of the women sporting
a billowing tablecloth in the vague shape of a dress.

I had to get out of watching any more of Xander stuffing
his face. "I am going to try to get in line for the buffet
before all the good stuff is gone, I will catch up with you two
later, maybe when you're less sweaty, Xander."

"Ha, Dr. Grant, don't count on that." Xander smirked as he
forked another mouthful down the hatch.

Kate took out another napkin from her purse and continued
patting Xander's forehead sweat. "Geez Louise, you are so
embarrassing, Xander. Dr. Grant, you should definitely get
something to eat before the buffet dries out, we will catch up
with you later. Maybe catch the fireworks together?"

"Sure, save me a seat."

I left towards the buffet. Those ribs really did smell
great. Something about charring sugar and pork in the hazy
humidity made for a Siren song that drew its end at stacks of
white china. The buffet line was long. On one side was a line
of food, and the other was a mass of mass -- so many protuberant
bellies in so many styles. Some were overflowing over a low
belt; I guess keeping a low belt can offer the psychological
benefit of a numerically smaller waist size. Why not just belt
the pants off at the knees and claim a 22 waist while weighing
three hundred pounds? Others secured their pants on the other
side of their abdominal globe with a high belt, cinching pants
just underneath the nipples, attempting to blend the belly into
a lower wall of flesh curtained behind wide but anatomically
implausible long pants. Why else would someone five foot eight
wear pants sized 50W, 50L? Most of the females looked

impossibly pregnant - everyone from little chunkster girls to post-menopausal grandmas sported an eight month gestational paunch. All these bellies were swinging awfully close to the food. This buffet line didn't need a sneeze guard; it needed a belly guard to prevent bellybuttons from dipping into potato salad and pork ribs. As I stacked my plate with barbeque, I had to look around to see if any mayonnaise or BBQ sauce had been displaced from the food and smeared on any of the surrounding bellies. Thank God, only one rack of ribs was missing some sauce, and it looked like it was on a guy who was in a previously clean looking dress shirt, and not on the frayed smock of the old lady who looked like she was wearing the only article of clothing that still fit her triple XL size and who looked at least three days off from her last laundry day.

These obese people were obviously well-off country club folk - a mishmash of big time stock brokers, successful businessmen and women, management executives, lawyers and doctors, all with their families. So by appearances, they must dine on aged New York strips, lobster tails soaked in drawn butter and crème brulees on a daily basis and the weight is just another outward sign of prosperity. They're adopting the way of some bygone cultures where it is a status symbol to be overweight, as if to show "I have so much material success that

I can consume more than I need and wear my excesses in a massive
skin suit". It is no surprise to see overweight, affluent
people; extra money has to go somewhere, and why not use it to
get padded in luxurious, fat dense delicacies. But, the means
to obesity has to go deeper than just money, because on the
drive over to the club, as he is every day at the same exit off
the Eisenhower, there was this homeless guy pan-handling with a
sign that read: "No werk, no home, help, I am hungrey." I call
him Hobo Heavy. This guy is easily three hundred pounds.
Impressive for someone who claims homelessness, no money and
spends his days begging on the side of the road to relieve his
self-proclaimed hunger. Calories are calories, whether they
cost a hundred dollars a pound or if they are free in a trash
can outside a Burger King, whether they are put together by a
culinary school prodigy or slapped together by a high-schooler
at his after school job, whether eaten by someone in Hugo Boss
or by someone wrapped in newspaper sleeping under an overpass.
Many of my own patients are on public aid, and even as their
parents beg me for prescriptions for over-the-counter
medications to get Dollar Store Tylenol paid by the state or for
a note to the electric company to override stacks of unpaid
utility bills with some vague medical need to get their power
turned back on or wrangling free advice over the phone instead

of paying for an office visit because of their economic plight,
I can see that their stated lack of money has not prevented dad,
mom and kid from eating to such an excess that their extra
calories could sustain another person each. A common excuse is
that healthy food costs too much and junk is often the cheapest
meal available. Yes, the calories per dollar in junk food is
much higher, and there is a logic to maximizing calories per
dollar when dollars are limited, but in obesity, an inefficiency
of calories per dollar is not the problem. Buying a few less
calories per dollar should be preferable for most. Buying a few
thousand extra calories on top of the required daily calories
should be supplanted with simply buying the required daily
calories in better quality. Most people cannot turn down paying
just five dollars for one grease filled value meal, as being the
much easier way to meal plan. Instead of planning a meal from
ingredients to recipe, they can just pick a number off a well-
lit menu while idling in their car. The easy way is the lazy
way, and the worst way. You can feed a whole family with about
five dollars worth of potatoes, frozen veggies and ground beef
(shepherd's pie, beef stew, sloppy joes), and save about five
hundred calories per person. Water is the cheapest and lowest
calorie beverage around, drinkable and flowing freely from any
tap, but everyone will pay any amount to hydrate with the

elixirs of soda and juice. Sure, some fruits and vegetables can
be pricey, out of season especially, but so are diabetes
medicine and heart attacks, which are always in season with
obesity. Money is not a limiting factor in excess calories; not
giving a shit is what buys the calories.

I spent the rest of the day setting a personal record for
pork and corn-on-the-cob ingestion seated under the willow tree
off to the side of the main lawn. Today was one day for me not
to give a shit. I can't even imagine how some people live
eating like this every day. I was feeling bloated, nauseous,
and, periodically, a splash of bilious foodstuff would lip up to
the back of my tongue to give me a mucoid, acrid taste of what
was being slowly digested. My stomach can only digest what it
can per hour, and this load was way above its threshold, so
pounds of pork butt has to wait in line to get at my digestive
juices, intestines, colon and toilet. A punch to the stomach
would've burst me open like a piñata to spew half digested pig
out to all the partygoers. The obese must be able to push aside
these feelings of over-satiety, like a they do to bowls of
steamed organic vegetables, and just ignore the discomfort and
regurgitant to keep on eating. The body has the defense of
discomfort to try to regulate maximal intake, but when those
defenses are ignored for so long, the body has to adapt by just

turning off the discomfort sensor, so the gullet gets a constant green light. My discomfort was making me feel so tired. It must be a way for the body to sleep through the worst of digestive overloading. This willow tree provided the perfect shaded spot to doze off this bomb of a meal. Plus, it was a great vantage point to watch the Xander show.

After that monster lunch, he took a long nap on a pool lounge chair, using two adjacent sun loungers to support his haunches. He snored loudly and stopped breathing a few times, only to jostle out of REM and resume sucking in air each time. When he finally awoke after two and a half hours, Xander wiped his mouth, rocked back and forth to get momentum off the sagging lounge chairs, and strolled back to the buffet to spend the next few hours trying to eat another whole pig by himself. He also started wearing down the grass in between the buffet and bar to continually fill his plastic cup at the keg. Beer seemed to be his new breast milk. Now he was tanked up with the smoked meat of two pigs and a full pony keg. He was exactly like when he was a baby, happily guzzling calories through unintelligible babbling, though now he was feeding himself and peeing in bushes. He had discovered another easy way to down a few hundred extra calories every day with minimal effort. And if he becomes like most people, he will never think of alcohol as calories, just as something to drink for good times. When he goes back to college in the fall, he'll start packing on the pounds exponentially quicker while eating the same diet and wonder why. His fat will become more concentrated about his abdomen, and he'll start joking that his pot belly was becoming a keg. Never to blame weekends spent at frat parties and bars. Then when he grows older, he will never blame the happy hour drinks or the post-dinner cocktail or the twelver while watching the Bears vs. Packers. Unless the drink is made from a blended bacon cheeseburger, its calories will never count in Xander's mind.

Dusk was now settling in quickly, and the Xander show was winding down. He was stumbling around the lawn, sloshing his beer from his plastic cup, shirt untucked with sweat saturated around the collar and both armpits, and swiveling his pumpkin head from side to side looking for his parents, his head seemingly sitting directly on his sternum, as any neck was long engulfed by the thick scarf of fat wrapped around jawline to chest.

"Mom, where the balls are you sitting, when are the fireworks freakin' starting?" Xander was literally shouting. His chest mass insulating his lungs and vocal cords created a cave effect which made his voice bellow as if sounded by the combined echoes of a dozen spelunkerers.

Kate ran up to him and started steering him towards their seats near the lake. She grabbed his arm, and as she speedily backpedaled to lead him, I could see the brisk pace was starting to nauseate him. Xander's face tensed briefly, he grabbed for his mouth, and then he vomited all over Kate's frontside, the spaces between his sausage fingers having formed a series of small nozzles that caused a wide spraying of vomitus onto her chest rather than the typical no-handed upchuck of one thick sloppy brushstroke. I guess pork, barbeque sauce and beer make for something that looks like diarrhea. Kate's white dress shirt was a clean canvas to display this Pollock of gluttony. Her breasts were really evident now, but this was one awful wet T-shirt contest. Kate took a few steps, grabbed for her mouth, then proceeded to form hand blinders and direct a stream of vomit onto a patch of lawn in between two families of picnickers; it looked like she had drunk her share of strawberry daiquiris. Albert rushed in and rescued them both. He grabbed them by the arms and ran them away from their bile soups, somehow without vomiting himself, though he dry-heaved a few times. The whole Xander family was now disappearing over the grassy hill and towards the parking lot.

They missed a great fireworks show.

PARK BENCH

Running has to be the worst activity ever. Propelling
oneself for the sake of propelling oneself is idiotic. I feel
like crap during the entire run - a little lightheaded, eyes
blurry from sweat, nose and throat filled with a slurry of spit
and snot, chest burning, nipples chafing, stomach cramping, sore
butt and thighs, noodle-y legs, shin splints, and achy arches.
Then I feel great when it's over. I guess I have to do it
because my masochistic body tells me it's good for me. I
anticipate today being no different: feeling awful for forty
minutes, then getting a wave of satisfaction for pushing my body
past some self perceived limit. I guess some of the high has to
do with the fact that I'm pre-paying the penance for the
chocolate shake I'm going to have after dinner tonight. Cave

men always stayed in shape from needing to run everywhere to catch food. I have to run to get rid of food.

I usually run near a park by my house. It is a pleasant patch of grass; usually there is some little league game stirring and some dogs chasing Frisbees and some pretty girls dozing on their backs getting some sun. Usually a sure bet for some great scenery to keep my mind off how much I hate running. But, not today.

It looked like Xander and Xander's twin wearing a long blonde wig were sucking face on a park bench. They looked like they were frantically trying to climb to the top of each other. They both had asses in the front and back. It was a squash humping a gourd.

I am sure Xander got sick of being alone. Every male starts out thinking he can sex Heidi Klum. Movies always have some awkward geek being able to win over a gorgeous woman with just his sparkling decency and uniqueness. Hell, *Knocked Up* had Seth Rogen sexing Katherine Heigl. But then, as the rejections start to add up in the real world due to physical or financial or personality status issues, Heidi starts to become Tara Reid to your friend's mom to Jill the Burger King girl. Xander must've got fed up with putting lipstick on his left hand and calling that his girlfriend or spending hours searching and downloading internet porn so he could use his robotic vagina simulator in front of his computer screen. So he hit upon this girl, and decided to take it.

Regardless of who the woman was, Xander is lucky; women are more tolerant of big bodies than men. Fat chicks have to accept being tossed aside or start getting really slutty, irrespective of their personality, just to make it with the typical male sensibilities. And they will likely never be considered the dream girl; at best, just an okay-for-now-while-I'm-drinking-and-horny girl. Fat dudes only have to worry about trying to attract a girl with their status, money or personality, and not so much their physique. No amount of money and status will get Rosie a spot on *People*'s "50 Most Beautiful" list, but a little paunch has never hurt Russell Crowe with the ladies; a few pictures of a heavier Jessica Simpson get national coverage while a pudgy Val Kilmer in swimming trunks gets placement at the bottom left on page thirty surrounded by blown up pictures of a possibly cottage-cheese thighed Tyra Banks. Fat men can become successful and earn the option to shoot for the stars and see what they can hit; fat women usually have to take whatever they can get given their present deviation from society's stereotypical image of attractiveness, regardless of moneyed status. Pavarotti's ladies were beauties with bodies; Rosanne got Tom Arnold. Xander was no Pavarotti, and was probably about double that tenor's size. His body would test even the most tolerant of women. Yet he still found one.

Even for him, food was not enough to satisfy everything. He got to this body size because, for a long while, he got off on eating so much that it far superseded the pursuit of any sensation that he could have gotten by putting his flesh into a warm, soft, wet orifice. Someone that has worked to blow up to over three fifty does not have attracting the opposite sex as a high priority. If Xander thought humping a cooling Bananas Foster felt as good as eating it, he would be much trimmer. Even in movies, crotching a pie was not sweet enough to stop the pursuit of sexing a real female. The need to feed his simmering sexual starvation eventually grew to an extent that it won out over his need for gustatory overindulgence. A love of food gave him the weight, and the weight made him tired at recess, tired walking to class, tired walking at graduation, tired walking up office steps, tired walking to the buffet, and eventually tired of walking alone.

This current scene at the park only proves the adage (my adage) that save for the odd fetishist, the obese usually come in pairs - similar to intra-sexual insects, wherein only they will tolerate mating with someone that may potentially eat them.

Go to any family dining establishment and there will be plenty of families where clearly a three hundred pounder mated with another three hundred pounder and created little future three hundred pounders. Of course Xander himself was a new mutation, weighing as much as Kate and Albert put together, but if he is able to procreate with this girl, there will be another litter of Xander's born. She may be pregnant right now, she could be 8 1/2 months pregnant for all I know, but her girth makes it impossible to distinguish a bulge of abdominal fat from a bulge of fetal life. No one could comment for fear that their congratulations on a baby-to-be are instead congratulations on ingested Krispy Kremes. It could be that she does not even know if she was carrying a little Xander, ignoring nausea as a bad Big Mac and her lack of menses to her baseline metabolic dysfunction from obesity, leading to one day when she gets bad cramps after eating a full package of Oreos with a gallon of whole milk, then runs into the bathroom expecting to BM and instead comes a toilet baby.

Obviously they need to somehow have sex to create a baby. The usual simple task of insertion becomes a bastard task between morbidly obese persons and makes getting sperm to ova their miracle of life, rather than the actual birth of the baby. Mounds of flesh obscure genitals and create mushy obstacles that

necessitate superhuman angles to align penis and orifice.
Abdominal panni has to be lifted and moved aside, and rhythmic
movements make for an ever shifting plane, like trying to keep
an avalanche of mayonnaise from overwhelming a small pubic
village during an earthquake using just your hands. The physics
of obese intercourse are mind-blowing, but it must occur because
this park's playground is filled with their progenies; little
rolys taxing swings and monkey bars with faces smeared in
chocolate and hands sticky from earlier ice cream snacks. How
does a morbidly obese man's penis ever physically get into
morbidly obese vagina? How does sperm ever get to that egg?
Does the man fill a kiddie pool with ejaculate so the woman can
take a fertilizing squat? Or is it related to why my local
megamart is always selling out of funnels?

It looked like Xander and his lady were eating each other.
This was way too much tongue and heavy petting for a mid-
afternoon on a public bench. Both Xander and his lady were
wearing black T-shirts with "Fat is Beautiful" on the front in
block lettering. The tees were like every tee on the morbidly
obese, in that the bottom of the shirts were unable to get all
the way over the expanded belly and instead only able to stretch
near the apex of the protrusion, unable to fully cover the
hanging fleshy mass that was now flopped over their respective

groins. I knew those exact shirts from the Fat Awareness Club
that had a vocal membership at the nearby college, where I heard
Xander had enrolled a couple years ago. The shirts were their
uniform. This club always has cupcake giveaways most spring and
summer weekends on the town's sidewalks, yelling out "Fat is
Beautiful!" on megaphones while handing out the baked goods with
their "Fat is Beautiful" slogan in icing on the top and with
pamphlets attached espousing anti-fat discrimination bullets –
the latest pamphlet pushed into my hands had on it articles
titled "Would you call your grandmother a fatass?" and "Buddha
had a belly". The cupcakes were damn good, though; I didn't
expect anything less from true connoisseurs of sweets. The club
also had fundraising car washes a few times a summer with some
of their more topside voluptuous female members in bikini-tops
and flowing wraparounds as the sudsy spongers. It was a
militant obesity club – less about a support group to become
healthier than about forcing everyone to acknowledge their right
to be overweight and be considered beautiful. It was really
just a club of people that found it too hard to change their own
habits, so they were efforting to try to change everyone else.
Yes, it is an inalienable right to be fat, but it is an absurd
notion that people should be forced to behold another person's
idea of beauty. "True beauty is on the inside" -- that is empty

rhetoric everyone can get behind for show, but in actual practice beauty is a visual medium. No amount of cupcakes and megaphoning in slicked up size 20 bikinis fronting double D's are going to convince me that a three hundred pound woman in a purple miu-miu dipping bon-bons in drawn butter is the same as Victoria's Secret models slowly licking away lollipops. Beauty beholding is in itself also an inalienable right. That subjectiveness applies to everyone, regardless of girth: I think Kate Moss looks closer to an alien than a supermodel, but my college roommate stickied every picture of her he could get in his left hand. It isn't that the world is filled with shallow people, as much as that theorem is used as reason for obese self-loathing, it is that people are evolutionarily hardwired to be attracted to their perceived versions of healthy people. The chances of producing future generations during harder times was exponentially smaller if someone was unable to move fast enough to catch food or chronically sick with organic diseases or dead decades before healthier peers.

Xander apparently views any mate as healthier than loneliness, and that mutated axiom made this overfilled bag of wet laundry irresistibly arousing. He couldn't stop his hands from fondling the mounds of flesh underneath every letter of the silk-screened slogan on the front of this girl's T-shirt. He

was also fondling every inch of her backside, which had every
bit of full breasts as her frontside, made from the pouching of
excess skin over her scapulas. These back breasts were equally
engorged in fat cells and glandular mass, but were never going
to nourish any infant.

I am reminded of a charity dinner I attended recently for
the local children's hospital at Morton's, which was emceed by
the very attractive local 5 o'clock news anchor and her new
husband. I remember them sharing a quiet moment at their table
after her duties were done, and exchanging a few loving kisses
and caresses. Very sweet. Xander pawing at neck rolls, with
his hands occasionally disappearing into skin flaps, while he
received a dry handjob by getting his front-ass rubbed by
overstuffed sausage fingers was criminally indecent. PDAs
should be better regulated by law for the sake of society's
mental health; no one wants to see Jabba suck face with Grimace.

Full breasts were on both Xander and his lady, and both
sets blended on top of bellies into mounds of flesh
indistinguishable from ass. Man should be distinguishable from
woman by the existence of breasts in the least - even "A" cups
perked under a shirt have the distinct silhouette of a woman's -
but breasts in these two had long disappeared into androgynous

wormholes of adipose. Breasts, back-ass, front-ass, and
genitals all disappeared into flaps of fat.

Kate has great breasts - a supple palm-full withperfectly
proportioned areolas and reactive nipples. I enjoyed their
every benefit in high school. She started out as a little fat
girl in grade school that would pass on playing outside to eat
donuts in front of cartoons, but after years of her brothers
calling her King Kong Kate, she went vegetarian for a while in
junior high and became a gym rat. She got slender and fit just
in time for high school. Lucky for her, the weight didn't come
off her chest. Lucky for me, too. As an added bonus, she still
held twinges of the self-esteem of a fat girl. Low self-esteem
at an age where making a boy happy makes self-esteem? I didn't
know it at the time, but that was how a scrawny geek like me
snagged her back then. Though that ended in a sour flash. The
last time I saw her breasts in the flesh was at the start of
senior year: me walking into a laundry room at a party, Kate
topless, on her knees, in front of a pant-less James Keene. At
least she married the next guy she went out with after dumping
James a couple weeks later.

I am feeling nauseous from this run.

Xander brought his dog to park too. This little guy was
tied up to the corner of the bench, seated contently in the

grass, checking out the scene out at the park while his master was porking. This puppy was panting heavily. Out of breath from sitting. He was a Sharpee, all extra skin and rolls, but also was an overweight Sharpee, so he looked like a furry Xander. This guy looked like one of those dogs that would keep eating whatever food he could get into his paws; fill a bowl with a cup, he'll eat a cup, fill it up with two cups, then two cups gone, spill a bag of Iams, better buy another bag tomorrow. I'm sure he was getting a ton of table food. Eating Xander's daily scraps would be a full meal in itself for any dog, but it looked like this furry guy was using it as a supplement to his dry dog food meal. The best hope for this dog would be if he got into a bad batch of dirt and snagged a tapeworm. Then maybe Xander will unknowingly pick up some infested doggie poop, contaminate his hand, then forget to wash up before dinner and eat a few sloppy joes seasoned with tape worm - instant weight loss plan. Then again, his calorie intake may overcome even the tapeworm, so all Xander would be left with is a fat ass tapeworm living symbiotically in his lower intestine.

Looks like Xander and his lady were leaving. Xander grabbed the leash off the corner of the bench with his left hand, patted his crotch downward and gave one of his lady's front boobs a playful squeeze with his right hand. They went off hand-in-hand down the sidewalk, two asses shifting side to side like a couple bean bag chairs on a see-saw. They were no doubt en route to his house to advance their play to the next level; flaps slapping on top of a stressing mattress finishing in a pile of sweaty, sticky flesh.

Hey, it's been forty minutes. That went by quick. The best part of the workout is right now, when the body is recovering in endorphins with the memory of the comparatively extended discomfort still fresh. Thank god, I am done for today.

Thank you, Xander.

BIG HOSPITAL

Doctors get sick too. They are terrible patients. They
know too much medicine and can play armchair quarterback with
every decision made by the medical staff. I am a terrible
patient.

I got a bad stomach bug from some kid I saw at the office
who spent the entire visit directing coughs into my mouth every
time I opened it to talk, and so I urinated from my colon for a
couple days straight. I got a little lazy in my hydration,
mainly because I could barely muster the strength to get out of
bed, much less keep drinking Gatorade, so I started falling
behind in my fluid replacement. My sister came to check on me
on the third day of my illness after a phone call with her where
I barely made sense - she said I was talking how my old stuffed
bear was scratching at my door wanting to borrow a cup of honey

and a can of tuna -- and when she tried to help me to the
bathroom, I passed out face down onto tile. Next thing I know,
I'm laying in a hospital room with an IV in my arm. I'm feeling
much better now after getting a few liters of fluid, good enough
to be home, but the ER doc didn't feel comfortable letting me
go, even after I called him a wuss to his face, so I had to stay
overnight. And my roommate was a familiar fat guy.

Xander didn't look too good. He looked like an enormous
egg laying on a gurney, right down to the shade of white.   He
was definitely sleeping not as routine, but as a vitally needed
rest to heal.

When the nurse came in to change my IV bag, I whispered to
her, "What is going on with Xander over there?"

"Cellulitis. In between his rolls. Diabetic."

I nodded.

I can only imagine it started as just a little irritation.
Just a little redness from some of his overabundant skin to skin
friction. Then it progressed to a little fungal infection.
Here was someone whose every redundant flaps of tissue became a
nutrient rich petri dish for organisms that should normally only
be thriving on a pathologic athlete's foot. I can't even
imagine the stench he was emanating up close -- a two week old
dumpster raccoon decomposing in his folds. Sweat, scum, and

skin constantly rubbing on skin combined with the ignored task
of hygiene had to have made for some odor - it must've gotten
pretty cheesy too, and separating the rolls must've looked like
the mozzarella stringing behind after taking a slice of hot
pizza. That's fairly easy to treat initially, though - some
cream and maybe a soaped rag on a stick for preventive cleaning.
But Xander must've let it fester - maybe due to embarrassment,
maybe because it was so common a condition to him as to be
ignored - that the fungus ate away the skin, breaking down the
key barrier to keeping bacteria out of the body, and so a raging
staph infection settled in for laughs. Then add in that his
body is not in optimal shape to fight off bacteria because of
his diabetes, and Xander being laid up in a hospital for IV
antibiotics is no big surprise.

   "Is he doing okay?"

   The nurse nodded. "He's a lot better today. He was close
to getting transferred to the University Center when he came to
the ER a couple days ago, but the antibiotics seemed to have
turned him around. Maybe this will get him to lose some
weight."

   "Yeah, maybe."

   The nurse did have a point. What has a reasonably good
chance of getting a morbidly obese person back on a healthier

track? Some life threatening event related to their obesity: heart attack, stroke, diabetes-related amputation, or maybe even a skin infection gone crazy. They spend their lives daring death, and when it gets close enough to nip them in the heel, they might decide to snap back some sense. It is a bit of sad human nature that the normal course is to consume, consume and consume until the bubble pops; hopefully this skin infection is the bubble popping for Xander.

But, not likely. Smokers smoke through their tracheostomies, people still drink after liver transplants and Xander will go right into an Italian beef joint straight from the hospital after discharge. The only snap for him will be when the coffin lid is finally shut.

Change is the exception to the rule. When weight is a problem, it will always be a problem. Look at Oprah; she has always struggled with weight, and she still struggles with weight. And she has a personal trainer and personal chef. And she is a billionaire. And she is on TV every day being watched by millions of other women. If anyone was going to crack the case, if anyone had incentive to crack the case, if it was able to be cracked, it would have been Oprah. So she still has to fight the battle, with all its ups and downs, slims and wides.

The January issue of *People* magazine always highlights stories of successful weight loss, or inspiring follow-ups of the past season's contestants on *The Biggest Loser*, I guess to inspire readers to start the New Year striving to get fitter, but those stories of people winning the battle against obesity chronicle a lifestyle where eating and exercising have become a regimented, military-like schedule. Egg whites and wheat toast at 0700 hours, coffee with skim milk at 1030 hours, grilled chicken on spring greens with a tablespoon of balsamic vinaigrette at 1200 hours, an apple and 4 oz. of almonds at 1500 hours, fifty minutes of cardio and twenty minutes of free weights at 1700 hours, 6 oz. grilled miso salmon with a cup each of wild rice and steamed green beans, 4 oz. of red wine and a fat free chocolate pudding cup at 1830 hours. Maintaining a healthy weight for these obese people had become so foreign that it only became possible with rigid obsession. And the process to get to that point is obscenely painful: even on *The Biggest Loser*, where these people are on an isolated ranch with nothing to do but work out, eat right and lose weight, many weeks are a disappointment of weight loss and some even put up a weight gain – even the prospect of nationally televised failure and the potential to win two-hundred and fifty thousand dollars are sometimes not enough motivation to lose weight. I guess the

People human interest stories are trying to inspire that facing challenges can lead to a happy ending, though in trying to do so, those articles only show that winning the perpetual fight against morbid obesity is only possible with meticulously instituted change, and ultimately, the prize is simply the opportunity to continue fighting. The war is never won for most; the problem just never goes away completely.

Xander's main issue fueling his obesity is that he has never even shown up to fight. Not even when his joints turned to mush to make even walking an exercise in pain, or when he developed type 2 diabetes in his thirties, or even when he had to start strapping on a breathing mask every night to force air down his trachea while he sleeps because his neck fat was so obstructive to his upper airway that it was causing periods of apnea. And now he almost had lost a fight for his life from an infection facilitated by rolls of fat.

The nurse quickly went from my bedside to Xander's. She continued with her patient assessment at a brisk pace. She lifted up his bed sheet and then his gown to clean his abdominal dressings. I craned my head up and took a peek. Xander's belly looked like it had just taken the brunt of a savage slapping fight and then someone spilled peach jelly all over it. The nurse lifting and replacing Xander's gown sent a waft of his infectious gas towards me. It smelled like grocery store garbage left out in the summer sun for a few days. She stepped to the open door and signaled for help. Five burly orderlies walked in and settled around the bed sheet. They all grabbed a chunk of sheet and the nurse started a quiet count.

"One, two, three."

And with six grunts, the nurse and orderlies turned Xander about thirty degrees from his left side to his right. A corner of his gown snagged on a bedrail and flipped up towards his abdomen. There were no genitals visible, just hanging skin and thighs, with the nether regions buried in the netherworld underneath all that extra tissue. The nurse quickly flipped his gown back down, then readjusted pillows, sheets, and IVs. Then she shrugged. The orderlies nodded and left. A reasonably well performed production of "As Xander Turns".

The nurse stood back to examine her work. "Tomorrow is going to be a bitch."

"What's tomorrow?"

"He's going for a CT."

"Oh."

"The doctors don't think he's even going to fit in the machine. We may have to send him to the zoo."

Patient list for the Brookfield Zoo CT machine tomorrow: Grizzly Bear, Sperm Whale, Xander, and a baby Elephant. What the hell. I guess when you reach a point where simple medical imaging needs to be done behind the Pachyderm House, you don't give a crap about appearances too much. Being half naked in a XXXL hospital gown where half the staff has ogled your raging rolls of infection while marveling at disappeared genitals is comparatively the Mother Theresa of dignity.

The nurse wrote a few things down in Xander's chart and walked out the door. Xander started shifting a bit. Then he farted.

I have to get out of here.

Part of the reason I loathed to go to the hospital was the cost. This stay is going to cost me at least a few thousand dollars. If I could've just toughed out a few hazy and diarrheal days at home without risking death, I would have done it to save the cash. Why does it cost me, a healthy never before hospitalized patient, a couple thousand dollars to just get some fluids dripped into me? Looking over at Xander's face suck in air, his arm IV suck in fluids and antibiotics, and his mattress suck down towards the floor made me want to switch off his bed's brakes and shuffleboard him out of the hospital. I have to subsidize Xander. All of his semimonthly doctor visits to manage his diabetes, blood pressure and cholesterol, all of the times he says fuck it and eats an Italian beef and chili cheese fries instead of taking his insulin and wakes up in the Emergency Room, all of the times his comorbidities force the Emergency Room doctors to give him the million dollar heart attack workup for any chest pain because it would be malpractice to ignore the fact he is a morbidly obese diabetic, and now a two week stay to treat a skin infection caused by redundant skin and poor hygiene topped off with a trip to the zoo to get a damn CT scan have to be paid in part by people like myself. The cost of insuring Xander's medical care has to be shared, like how turning him in his hospital bed needed to be shared by the efforts of six people, or how I imagine his casket one day needing to be shared by a baker's dozen of pallbearers. Other people's premiums have to cover the potential cost of their own medical care as well as the losses from this guy's obesity-related, chronic medical issues. There is no way Xander's own insurance premiums could ever cover all of his medical care. This guy eats even health resources at such a rate to affect everyone's insurance premiums. People always rail against the government or insurance companies or doctors to blame them for the high cost of health care, but never is any connection made with McDonald's 1 billion served. Drinking too much, smoking too much and certainly eating too much cause most modern day health problems, and these are all preventable, but because people don't suffer instant morbid consequences from these habits, they continue to suck back tobacco, booze and grease, and eventually become train wrecks of failing health that suck down most of society's health resources. No one wants to look at themselves as the culprits to rising health care costs, they much rather blame some faceless corporation or system, so the underlying reasons of poor individual health decisions go unchecked and perpetuate.

For hospitals, Xander is a goldmine. A fat guy with a scrolling strap of chronic medical problems with good private insurance. The profit generated from his insurance company's good reimbursement rates for his numerous hospitalizations probably allows the hospital to absorb the losses from the capped reimbursements of a dozen public aid patients. Hospitals can count on the fact that once a morbidly obese person comes in with a complaint, the medical machinery has to get started and there is no release home until everyone is reassured that this person won't drop dead in the next few days. That always takes a few thousand dollars of tests.

But, it is not money spent to cure. That would be impossible. No amount of medicine will ever get the obese to become skinny without the active participation of the individual. Instead, it is a few thousand dollars of medical interventions towards the goal of just getting that fat guy off a runaway death train and back onto the more tolerable track towards early death at the slower pace of one fried chicken bucket at a time. That medically assumed eventual outcome is the reason no one is too surprised when someone morbidly obese needs medical attention, though sometimes the hamburger fed march towards death jumps ahead a few quicker steps at a time. Chest pain? Tell a doctor the sufferer is morbidly obese and the doc will think, "Hmmph, figures." Now doctor has to rule out a heart attack even though the pain is probably due to just eating four Arby's roast beef sandwiches drenched in horsey sauce. A little short of breath? Hmmph, figures. It could be a pulmonary embolus from massive gravity slowing his lower extremity circulation to the point of syrup, then tossing a few resultant clots to his lungs, so doctor has to spiral chest CT this guy, even though it's more likely just a fat guy sucking air from simple deconditioning. Back pain? Hmmph, figures. Better make sure this guy didn't crush a few vertebrae from his mass shifting in his sleep even though the pain is likely from his spine being maximally taxed supporting superhuman weights all day, everyday. Knee pain and can't walk? Hmmph, figures.

Lower legs are swelling? Figures. Getting pneumonia a few times a year? Figures. Boil on the ass? Figures. It doesn't matter what the ailment, obese persons getting sick are accepted as the norm, and death is known to be always hovering over their masses.

The next day, when I awoke, Xander was unsteadily shuffling to the bathroom with a couple orderlies and a nurse assisting him.

"Hey, Dr. Grant! How are you feeling?"

"Pretty good, Xander, how about you?"

"Much better today. I woke up today feeling as good as I have since I got here. Thought I'd try to walk to the bathroom today, but all these dang medicines they're giving me are messing with my balance."

It's always something else besides the obvious. Intravenous fluids and antibiotics causing a waddling gait? How about years of de-conditioning coupled with a few days of total immobility? Even the healthiest of patients will lose significant strength after being bedridden for a few days, so that deterioration will easily push someone morbidly obese into an invalid. In his mind, he was the victim of some outside agent's side effect. I guess that is easier to swallow than to realize that his deteriorating balance was self inflicted, that his deteriorating health was more suicide than manslaughter.

He was grunting with every step. "Dang, my legs are killing me. They're all swollen up and red with a rash, probably from all these toxins in my body trying to get out."

How about years of deconditioning and weight gain obliterating his lower extremity venous valve threshold? A combination of limited blood flow from a lack of activity and a constant massive downward pressure from excess mass have made Xander's legs swell up with extra fluid that got backed up from his taxed blood return system. Back flow is the simple diagnosis, rather than some self-created, abstract diagnosis of toxin expulsion. When the veins don't work, there's going to be alterations in oxygen delivery to tissues, including skin, and when some of that skin doesn't get enough oxygen, there's going to be damage and inflammation to that skin, and a resultant rash. That swelling and redness was directly fat-related whether Xander wanted to face it or not.

Xander disappeared into the bathroom with his trio of helpers. Almost everything that someone does in the bathroom should be able to be done alone - brushing teeth, showering, urinating, stooling - but once bathroom activities need assistance, it should be taken as a sign that something has gone terribly wrong. The sound of Xander's whistling "Somewhere Over the Rainbow" from the bathroom made me believe he was not taking it as that.   Taking a piss for him was no longer the normally private show; it had become a repeating performance for a participating audience of three who were only there because they were getting paid to be there.

There was a flush and the foursome reappeared. "Dang, my knees. I can't wait to be done with this medicine." He leaned on each of the orderlies with each step, letting the nurse drag his IV pole, and slowly got back into bed. That bed seemed to sink a foot when he climbed onto it. "Whew, I am tired. I'm going to grab some shut eye."

And he did. The only thing to wake him two hours later was the lunch tray. It was an impressive lunch tray. He had ordered a few meals. I compared what was on his tray to my tray of a turkey sub and green beans, and it looked like I had gotten the hospital Happy Meal. He took the napkin, tucked it into the collar of his gown, arranged his plasticware neatly to his left, then went to work. He was brutally efficient. Big bites, then fork to plate to snag another mouthful to bring up to lips just as the first mouthful chews were winding down, and then repeated in dizzyingly quick succession. The sunshine from the window

skewed into rapid fire glints by his working plastic. It was
strangely mesmerizing.

He paused after getting through half his food. "Ugh, this
food is disgusting." Then he kept on eating. All he left was
just a pile of empty plates. He dozed off soon after.

I flipped on the TV to kill some time. The Shawshank
Redemption was on. Unbelievable movie.

"These walls are funny. First you hate 'em, then you get
used to 'em. Enough time passes, you get so you depend on them."

Xander had his own prison. Xander was in the hospital
because of complications from his morbid obesity, yet was doing
nothing to prevent another admission. He was wallowing in his
excess weight. The life he knew of sitting all day, eating all
day and playing the victim all day was now preferable to the
possible life waiting for him after dieting and exercise.

I kept down my lunch and was feeling even better than I did
when I first woke up this morning, so I got discharged home
later that evening. Leaving this room imparted an odd sense of
approaching more living, as if I was running a bit further from
the reach of the Grim Reaper. Xander was still asleep when I
made my way out of the room. If it wasn't for his snoring, I
would've thought he was dead the way his body was flopped on the
mattress. He was still breathing. For now.

AU BON PAIN

"So you think he needs to get gastric bypass surgery?"

I ran into Kate on my day off while getting a chocolate
muffin and coffee at Au Bon Pain. After being coerced to sit
with her, and some mindless small talk, this is where the
conversation led. Xander is thirty-eight and his mommy is still
worrying about his weight. And she's still oblivious why he
weighs more than both his parents combined. But, now at least
he wants to do something serious about it.

"No doubt about it, Kate."

"He's tried Atkins, South Beach, Weight Watchers, he's
gotten prescriptions for Meridia and Xenical, emptied out the
Walgreens stock of Hoodia, HydroxyCut, Trimspa, and Alli, did
some diet where he ate these weird cookies all day, and he even

went to Mexico to buy some stuff which only gave him bad stomach cramps and which made him gain ten pounds."

Xander was desperate. Not desperate enough to do the one thing that will work over the long term – diet and exercise – but desperate enough to try anything in search of the easy shortcut. Everyone wants a quick fix and have their problems fixed with just a simple pill. They want to keep eating bacon cheeseburgers and drinking chocolate shakes every meal, then watch TV all day from their lazy boys and still lose weight by just taking a bunch of herbs in pill-form. Everyone wants to be that "after" on the weight loss infomercial: to start out as a slumped blob of adipose and then magically turn into a tanned, oiled tank of muscle. As if decades of body abuse should only take days to reverse. That is the real laziness of morbid obesity: the all-out effort to avoid the guaranteed successful solution that requires continual hard work, to instead pursue the failing fads that require minimal work. Xander is lazy.

"Albert and I sent him to an obesity center in Arizona we heard about, but he only came back fifteen pounds lighter with a tan."

Fat clinics abound like cancer or surgery centers, signaling obesity's prominence onto the medical stage. These clinics' advertisements saturating print, radio and television, point to the lucrative nature of obesity - a limitless patient population willing to try a never ending variety of treatments with an equally never ending drive to find an easier way to drop pounds.

There are more than enough obese in the populace to sustain the fraud of weight loss specialists that got Cs in high school and went to school in the comparative strip mall of medical education. Chiropractors are educated in open admissions schools that teach pseudoscience and marketing to anyone that is willing to pay their tuition, yet these snake oil salesmen still have the gall to market themselves as "doctors" purporting "natural" medicine while delving into areas where they have not had a sniff of appropriate training, where scientific evidence is seen as an unwelcome foreigner and where any bit of sugar coated nonsense they are able to concoct is dispensed as cure. These are people that make their living in the zone of anecdotes and placebo effect, and with so many targets to choose from to drive up the chance of independently random successes, they will continue to happily chicken hawk the ample supply of misguided weight loss seekers.

There are so many obese and the concept of weight loss has become so ubiquitously relatable that it has become a Nielsen ratings buster, able to drive a reality show about the ultimate fat clinic as competition, *The Biggest Loser*, to frenzied popularity as there are more and more fat people to tune in to NBC to admire even fatter people lose weight in impressive fashion, liken to how people will tune in to watch professional athletes. Fat clinics can be helpful to jumpstart weight loss, but unless someone can live at one of these centers all day every day, or at least stay for the necessary months to get their eating and exercise habits reprogrammed, these clinics are not going to be more helpful than watching a late night infomercial on a magic weight loss pill discovered by some sketchy looking "doctor" spewing nonsense while trying to look the part in a white labcoat.

"Sounds like he needs surgery. How much does he weigh nowadays?"

"Close to four fifty."

Almost as many pounds as cents for a Big Mac meal. "Wow, that really is heavy. That is surgery-heavy, Kate."

"Really? It's really come to that?" Kate took a bite of my chocolate muffin and then her eyes started welling. I looked around at the crowded bakery. If she starts bawling it's going to look like I'm breaking up with her.

"Last month I got gastroenteritis from some kid and had a week of bad diarrhea, and lost fifteen pounds, so maybe Xander can go to the local daycare and eat some dirty diapers?" Kate broke her frown and smirked a little. I continued, "Or he could do like my buddy who went on a medical mission trip to South America and got a tape worm, which dropped him about forty pounds. He kept it off for like six months because that wormy sucker in his intestine was resistant to most antibiotics. He died though. He looked great at his funeral."

Kate now sported a full-on smile. Lame jokes always hit her funny bone. "Okay, okay, but seriously, is this surgery going to hurt him?"

It will definitely hurt. Surgery is no joke; scalpels hurt, probes hurt, having instruments inside your insides hurt, healing hurts. Pain is not the question. The real question Kate should be asking me is: Does Xander need to risk death by surgery in order to avoid death by cheeseburger?

Healthy people can die from surgeries. Iron Man competitors can die from surgery. Death is a baseline risk of any surgery, from simple face lifts to brain tumor excisions. But, performing major abdominal surgery on someone morbidly obese? Russian roulette. The obese are terrible candidates to have any surgery done to them; they are sedentary, resulting in poorer cardiovascular and pulmonary baseline functions, and likely with pre-existing co-morbid conditions like diabetes and

hypertension. Even routine procedures like finding a vein for
an IV, securing an airway or even listening to the chest with a
stethoscope are made exponentially more difficult due to the
respective obscuring, obstructing and muffling properties of
massive amounts of fatty tissue. It is a desperate point to
reach where the risks of surgery is far outweighed by the health
risks of letting someone continue eating and living status quo,
where invasive surgery becomes the most viable option to prevent
death by cheeseburger. It seems like gastric banding and
gastric bypass surgery should be rarer and more obscure
procedures. It is not - it's pop culture. People in the third
world must marvel at our continual access to massive amount of
food and shake their heads at the extent of medical care
available to treat the condition of overeating, as they sit in a
thatch hut recovering from malaria and about to eat a bowl of
plain rice as their only meal of the day. So, does Xander need
to risk death by surgery to avoid certain death by cheeseburger?
Undoubtedly, yes.

"Kate, it will be painful and risky, but it's better than
Xander never being able to feel anything, ever, because he's
dead from a heart attack."

Kate flinched just barely at the word *dead*. "I guess you're right. He doesn't have much of a life as it is now." Kate's frown had returned and she stared off blankly.

No doubt his weight has now put him in solitary. He was unable to walk more than a few steps before searing back pain necessitated a rest, unable to brush his teeth without breaking out in a sweat, having to use a cane to maneuver around even in his small bedroom, loathing to go out in public unless absolutely necessary because he feels people's stares and hears their murmurs. The amount of calories he needed to consume to maintain his weight had probably become so massive that most of his waking hours were spent eating or preparing for eating. Xander has hit a state where he needs someone to cut into his abdomen and reconstruct his gastrointestinal tract to purposely limit and malabsorb food because he can't put down that Twinkie on his own. There are so many horrible diseases that manifest as anorexia and malabsorption, but Xander needed to be surgically put into that state to counteract his excesses.

The really unfortunate thing was that he had a lot going for him. He had started some internet electronics company in college and was quite successful. He easily became a multimillionaire in his twenties. He bought his parents a huge house in a tony suburb and he built a custom ten thousand square

foot mansion on some land neighboring Michael Jordan's. He is a
member of the boards at the local Children's hospital and the
Art Institute, and has given away ten percent of all his
earnings to charity every year since making it big. He had even
been able to put his friend's dad into Washington by funding the
his Senate run last year. Xander was a big fish in this big
pond. Unusual for a fat, lazy guy, right?

Nope. Xander is only lazy about his weight, not lazy
about everything. There is a bad characterization that all fat
people are lazy. That absolutely cannot be true, because fat
people crowd every workplace, every square inch of society's
fabric, and if they were all lazy, the western world would
literally come to a halt. Reports would not get filed due to
Little Debbies, people would call in sick all the time due to
ice cream benders, and stores would close from 11-3 every day
just to ensure adequate time for the lunch buffet. Fat people
are not lazy in all aspects of their lives. It is quite easy to
work and eat simultaneously. But, the characterization
persists, and it probably arises from the stereotypical picture
of a lazy person: mouth agape on the couch, watching TV,
cushions molded to ass from hours of sedentary living, with
chips crumbs and soda cans everywhere. And that lazy person is
always fat. Living lazily can make you gain weight, but gaining

massive amounts of weight does not necessarily make you entirely lazy - only lazy about your health and well being. It's just an unfortunate consequence that being lazy about that one aspect of life creates such a large billboard to advertise that fact. Because Xander's obesity became a bare-breasted stripper advertising a $300 million dollar lottery jackpot of a highway billboard, people were going to slow traffic and bend fenders in noticing, and in their eyes, his exterior superseded everything industrious about him. All his capacity for hard work and his monetary successes became a footnote. That perception, and Xander's perception of that perception, is what made his reality now. He spent most days alone in his estate, eating away his money.

"Kate, I know he will be happier when he loses weight and can start living a more active life. There's a world out there that he can't access right now because of his weight."

She took another bite of my chocolate muffin. "He used to be so full of life, and now…"

Sure Xander was always fat, but now he was a human dirigible. Escalated morbid obesity. A difficult life made impossible. How did it get to this? Xander did what everyone does when their lives stabilize: they settle into comfort. Slim-fit low-rider jeans become elastic-banded, high-waisted sweats, crisp poplin shirts turn into one favorite threadbare T-shirt, clean shaven gives way to a Unabomber beard. It feels good to eat cheesy beef sandwiches and mozzarella sticks, it is comforting to down chocolate cake and whole milk in front of mindless TV every night, and a good cheeseburger and fries is pure happiness. It sucks to run on a treadmill and feel like throwing up for a half hour, it's really hard to pass on a few warm chocolate chip cookies, and feeling hungry feels like an alien sucking the life from belly. Eating and vegging out become the delusion of feeling well rather than the real wellness that comes from exercising and eating well. Life begins to be about what is comfortable rather than what is good for you.

I saw him one time at Baker's Square picking up a couple pies. Most people when they see someone pick up a couple pies assume it is for guests at a party. When people see Xander pick up two pies, they think it must be that night's dessert portion, and they shake their heads. Xander must've known that was what people were thinking because he came in head down, mumbled his order, paid quickly and shuffled out with his pies. I knew the pies were for a dinner party at his parent's house the next night, because I had been invited, though I also saw him eat the entire Oreo cookie pie for dessert at that party.

Ever eat a full pie for dessert? Or even half a pie? As difficult it is to maintain great physical fitness, it is equally as difficult to maintain massive weight. Eat six thousand calories a day? Ten thousand? Thirty-thousand? I have seen Xander eat an entire X-large pizza and wash it down with a 2-Liter of Pepsi. Kate has told me he spends thirty dollars at McDonald's for a dinner for one. I have seen Xander picnic in the park with a lunch of sandwiches measured by loaves of bread and packs of meat. It is a serious commitment to stay large. A rigid regiment needs to be followed and strictly adhered. First, ignore the fact that the quantity being eaten is multiples of even the excess portion sizes that the average person consumes -- four extra value meals for lunch, why not? Second, eat only high calorie concentrated grub -- don't waste valuable chewing on just a single patty burger when a triple stack can be stuffed into the mouth with just a little more effort. Third, eat all the time -- any period not spent eating is calories lost and calories that need to be made up to maintain massive weight. Burger King run at midnight, don't think about it, just do it. And lastly, stop caring and start justifying -- spiral into self-loathing and play the victim if necessary, to square away laziness and shirking personal responsibility in the mind.

Kate snapped back from her stare, and started crying. "Stupid genes we gave Xander! Stupid slow family metabolism! He had no chance from where he came from!"

I patted Kate's head as she cried, but this was ridiculous. Trying to blame obesity on a uniquely slow metabolism or a bad genetic inheritance is ridiculous. Metabolism and genetics are varied, but the road to morbid obesity is single: intaking multiple-fold calories than burned. Why can't anyone just admit that obesity is created from conscious decisions to intake a perpetual tsunami of excess calories? Deciding to make snack-size into party-size? Deciding to trade the Happy Meal for a Super Sizer? Deciding to be active for nothing more than just the goal of getting to the next meal? Intaking a week's worth of fats in one day, then de-conditioning the body to the point of becoming more slug than man, will certainly slow the metabolism, but that slowing has nothing to do genes - it's just the inevitable consequence of poor habits.

Obese parents have obese kids because they pass on their poor eating habits, and not because of some abstract fat gene. Kate and Al were lean and athletic, so her claim of some fat gene was even more absurd. Even if reality was suspended, and Kate and Al each had some unexpressed recessive fat gene they each gave to Xander, that genotype is still just a starting point, and it has nothing to do with why he is unable to improve on his phenotype. Not everyone is going to look like Brangelina, but that does not mean a life of never taking showers and always getting bad haircuts. Obesity is not a hopeless genetic mutation. Xander has decided to worsen perfectly adequate genetics with terrible behaviors. Now he has his mom buried in guilt.

Kate kept blubbering. "He's tried everything and worked so hard at his weight for so long, but his body just won't react."

As if claiming that nothing more could've been personally done for his weight loss was believable. Talking about working hard is not the same as working hard. Reading self help diet books is not the same as being on a diet. Buying an elliptical trainer is not the same as exercising. After cutting through all the self pity and excuses, there is just hard work. The hard work of weight loss is to just figure out a way to burn more calories than you eat. Simple. That extra three hundred pounds is not due to some special medical condition. It is due to the condition of gluttony. An entirely selfish condition. Playing the victim is the most pitiful means to skirt responsibility. A victim is someone that gets shot during a robbery or someone who invested with Madoff; there is no victim when someone finishes an entire black forest cake in one sitting

or decides to have an after dinner snack of a triple Whopper.
There is only obvious consequence.

I remember when Xander thought eating a bowl of oatmeal
every morning for breakfast would be the magic ticket for weight
loss. He caught me at the grocery store one day and revealed
his plan, rambling on about fiber and less fat absorption and
other generic nonsense he probably read in a a blurb on some
random website -- he must've forgotten I was a doctor and not
some housewife at a book club willing to take hearsay medical
knowledge as fact. He ate plain oatmeal every morning for a
month, and was puzzled that the scale wasn't budging. It was a
good thing that he was substituting oatmeal for his usual
breakfast of a packet of bacon and carton of eggs, but all he
did was prune a couple leaves when the entire tree needed to
come down. Never mind his triple value meal lunches, and King-
sized candy bar snacking, and full extra large pizzas for
dinners with entire French Silk pies for dessert, and midnight
runs to Taco Bell for bedtime snacks. He quickly went back to
his usual breakfast bombs. Fads like that are never
sustainable.

Massive weight gain is a consequence that can easily be
foreseen and expected from excessive eating behaviors; it is not
a cryptic puzzle unable to be logically prevented. The obese

put too much effort into the search for a magic decoder that will unlock the mystery of weight loss, when simple logic is to eat less. Living that simple logic may be difficult, but just because it is difficult does not mean it cannot be done or that it should not be done. "Why" is not the appropriate question. Someone that gets HIV from sharing heroin needles during whacked out weekend benders cannot wonder why. Taking down a whole deep fried chicken for lunch and then complaining about a five pound weight gain at the end of the week needs a shutting up. Kate, shut up about Xander.

I reached into my pocket and pressed my speed dial. I called my pager. Katie was still tearfully musing about Xander. The anticipation was making my stomach churn, as if I had eaten a bag of White Castle washed down with a gallon of chocolate milk, or what Xander would call a little bite. How long does it take to go from wireless station to radio signal? My pager finally went off.

"Damn, it's the hospital. I am so sorry Kate, but I have to go. Hey, don't worry so much, he'll get on the right track after surgery, I just know it."

I gave Kate a hug.

When a woman is crying, I will say almost anything to slow the tears. I told my ex-wife at a wake that her mother was a

super nice lady, even though her mother's soul was black tar.
Xander is not going to get on the right track after surgery. I
get the feeling everyone thinks surgery is going to be an
instant cure-all, and that Xander is going to be the next *People*
magazine cover story of victorious weight loss. Surgery is just
a band-aid until Xander can learn to control his weight alone.
That control is never happening. No amount of time bought under
a knife is ever going to quell his need to gorge. He is a food
dumpster.

I broke the hug, my arm brushing her right breast at
release, and then I rushed out the door into the fresh, fresh
air.

ADJUSTMENTS

Taco Bell Fridays. I really looked forward to my Friday
nights, which nowadays consisted of picking up a chili-cheese
burrito and three hard shell tacos from the Bell, sitting in
front of my flat screen and watching whatever until I fell
asleep on the couch. It was just a great way to unwind from a
week of work, at least for someone my age. It was unwinding
after having to deal with entitled parents all day and having to
give the same schpeel ad nauseam trying to explain why every
sniffle or sore throat doesn't require antibiotics and then
having them leave in a huff that they didn't get what they
wanted.   To have to deal with parents that think they know more
about medicine than someone who went through med school and
residency and years of practice and hundreds of hours of CME
because those parents read some stuff on the internet or heard

something from some other non-physician family member. After
spending my week dealing with those parents, I always choose
downtime activities that require no contact with any people.

This Friday, the drive-up was crazy, so I decided to park
it and walk into the restaurant to get my order. I caught
myself at the world "restaurant". Taco Bell being called a
restaurant? Like a bowler being called an athlete. It is not a
restaurant when the menu only consists of the same seven
ingredients mixed and matched in slightly different
combinations.

"Hey, Dr. Grant!"

The voice jolted me. It was Xander. He was seated by
himself near the back window. He looked a little bit slimmer.
I walked over towards him.

"Hey, Xander, how are you doing?"

"Great, really great. Are you making a run to the border
like me?"

"Yeah, just picking up some dinner. I love this place."

"Me too. It's a shame I can't eat as much of it anymore."

I looked down at his tray and it had just three hard tacos
on it.

"Oh yeah, your mom mentioned you might get surgery. How's
it been going?"

Patting his belly, "Not too bad. I've lost twenty pounds in the last three weeks, so that's pretty good."

"That's great, Xander. You look good."

"Thanks, doc. I went with the gastric banding. I'm getting so full, so fast now. But, I have to keep going into the doctor's office to get it retightened."

"Well, that's just the process."

"But when I first had to get my band retightened, I felt full after only a few bites for a while, then I starting feeling hungry even with more and more food, so then had to get it retightened again."

"You should tell your doctor about that."

"I did, but all he told me was that I have to use some willpower. Hell, if I had willpower, I wouldn't have needed the band."

I laughed. It was a funny point. Misinformed, though. Anyone can eat through their banding if they don't try to make any changes. The band surgically shrinks the stomach and that smaller stomach gets full faster, but the feeling of that artificial satiety can be overridden, just as the normal feeling of satiety was overridden for so long to eliminate the sensations of normal satiety and unleash the abnormal obesity that required the banding. When that override happens, food backs up and the esophagus becomes the extension of the stomach. Like sewers becoming full and backing up into the pipes of your home. It's called overpacking the pouch.

"Xander, unfortunately, the band is not the end-all cure-all for obesity. It's just a band-aid until you can figure out how to regulate your own food intake. It'll help you in the short term, but if you don't work at controlling your diet, even the band won't fix everything for the long term."

"Yeah, I guess you're right, Dr. Grant."

"Hey, three hard tacos is a decent portion. You're doing okay. Are you exercising?"

"Not yet, my back hurts too much. Even walking kills."

That pain is the body trying to hold onto being sedentary. Of course it's going to hurt when you're a blob trying to transition from sedentary to active. It's supposed to hurt. It's supposed to be hard. Or else everyone would be running marathons instead of gorging on marathon buffet sessions every day. That's part of the reason so many fall deeper into obesity - because it's hard to stay in shape. It requires daily effort with negligible immediate benefits and with no real end. On a day to day basis, running a few miles and eating healthy doesn't feel any better than ice cream and a nap, so it becomes easy to slide out of shape. Most daily activities just require the ability to sit on a chair for long periods of time, so the sneaky loss of physical fitness will not be noticed because the body is never cardiovascularly taxed to test its limits. If that daily maintenance is neglected, the work of staying in shape accumulates, and soon it becomes a mountain. The cumulative massive effort it now takes to overcome that mountain in the way of changing from an obese slug into a fit machine, only makes the benefits and end seem further away, so the defeatist mind sets in and the effort never get undertaken and instead the mountain just gets bigger.

Looks like Xander had his food plumbing reorganized just so he could stay sedentary and still lose weight. His fat ass is half-assing it again. Sure, any movement away from morbid obesity is technically getting healthier, just as eating a Big Mac meal with a diet coke is technically healthier than a Big Mac meal with a chocolate shake, but the ultimate goal is to be healthy and just getting skinnier is not always healthier. Runway models that strut Versace and Prada are certainly skinny, but they likely exist on diets of cigarettes and caffeine. Women on the covers of *Cosmo* and *Redbook* always look fit and shaped with lean muscle, though they're helped with botox, a pre-photo shoot crash diet and photoshop. *Men's Health* displays a cut-up freak of a muscled tank on its cover monthly, suggesting him as an example of the possible results of following its articles espousing the best diet and workout tips, but he likely just finished a cycle of performance enhancers and has a costume of a body with bad acne on his unseen back, a catalog of damaged internal organs and shriveled peas for testicles. Too much is Hollywood magic. Hollywood owns the image of attractiveness and it is a skinny one, regardless of fitness. Everyone wants to be attractive at some level, so people try to look slim at all faddish costs. Eating only meat doused in butter and equating Wonder bread to poison? Drinking nothing but maple syrup, cayenne and lemon juice for two weeks? Using a stainless steel tube to suck fat out of an incision like a wet-vac cleaning up drunk vomit? Everyone wants a shortcut to the appearance of health. There is none. But, because of frank laziness, the goal has become only about looking superficially healthy rather than doing the work to actually be healthy.

"Well, you have to start exercising. Just start real light, like stretching or even walking for five minutes at a time, then if you can do that, then try ten minutes, then fifteen, then you can keep slowly increasing your activity and intensity so you'll be running a marathon in no time."

Xander laughed, "Me running a marathon? That's crazy."

"It's not crazy. Losing weight is great and all, but you should really be focusing on getting healthy. It is very possible to be fit and still be a little overweight, just like it is possible to be out of shape and really skinny."

"Really?"

"Who do you think is healthier: a skinny guy that sits on his ass all day, or a chubby guy that just ran the Chicago marathon?"

"I hear what you are saying, but it's also hard to find time to exercise; I'm so busy with my business sometimes."

"How many dinners have you skipped this week because you were too busy?" I looked down at Xander's tacos.

"Um, none, I guess."

"If you can set aside thirty minutes every day to eat, you can set aside thirty minutes to exercise."

"Yeah, I guess you're right, doc."

"It's just priorities. What do you prioritize more, eating or exercising? If you're obese, the priorities need to be flipped."

"Yeah." Xander took a bite from his last taco and chewed slowly, letting his teeth and saliva disintegrate the bite into mush before sending it down to his pouch.

"Diet without exercise is like that taco without the shell."

Xander laughed as he popped the last bit of the taco into his mouth. "You're right, doc. Man, you are right."

I am right. It's good advice. Not many people will use busy schedules or stressful days or being too tired as reasons to completely skip meals consistently. Most will drop what they are doing at almost any cost when they are hungry to grab a quick bite of anything - even if it is just miscellaneous meat in a fried corn-like shell topped with iceberg shreds and cheesy strings.

That taco without a shell metaphor could be dripping with a little bit of personal hypocrisy, though. Here I am, tossing advice about diet and exercise at a Taco Bell, just before I am about to eat three tacos and a burrito, which I have eaten almost every Friday for a few years now, and just before I then go home and not move from in front of the TV for hours. I am giving all that advice even though pizza is my absolute favorite food, of which I will eat three-fourths of a large deep dish pie every sitting, with cold leftovers for the next morning's breakfast, at least once a week. And I eat at least one chocolate covered something every day, most days it being chocolate covered chocolate in chocolate sauce. And I can never turn away from a well-crisped basket of fries. Doctor heal thyself? A good thought, only I don't need healing. This is

not hypocrisy because no one is demanding perfection, just
moderation. I may have some bad dietary habits, like any
average guy (a life never eating fries or chocolate is no life
to me), but I don't let those habits ruin the rest of my life -
I force myself to work out hard four times a week, mix in some
salads before dinners, pass on the donuts most mornings and will
stop at three-fourths of a pizza rather than downing a full one
by myself. So I have been able to stay healthy through the
years. Admittedly, it has taken more effort as I have gotten
older, but it's what I have to do for my health so I do it. The
fact that my less than ideal eating habits can still be part of
a sufficiently healthy lifestyle just goes to show how far from
moderation someone has to go to get morbidly obese. If someone
can maintain relative health even with mediocre eating habits,
let them be, but if eating habits become problem eating habits
as shown by massive weight gain, then it's time to shuttle
current habits and change. But that potential change is too
much of an obstacle for most people - it becomes a horrifying
prospect to have to overcome terrible eating habits ingrained by
obese parents since childhood who allowed Little Chunky to eat
whatever in whatever quantity, to overcome comfort food being
set as McDonald's and Twinkies, to overcome the lifestyle of
having daily activity barely rising above inanimate object

status, or to overcome the anticipated discomfort of the regular cardiovascular exertions needed to maintain health. But, they have to be overcome. And that is all doctors are trying to get across when harping about diet and exercise: just care about your health the right way.

I had a colleague in residency named Barry that weighed over three hundred pounds. His white coat looked like a bed sheet. Yet, his patients never laughed in his face when he told them they were overweight and offered advice on how to lose weight. That was because he always gave his standard lecture on portion control and exercise with self-depreciation and in a tone that he was giving the advice with only their best interest at heart. Barry was just trying to get them to care about their health, even though he wasn't caring too well for himself. I guess his patients still figured the advice was good, regardless of whether the giver followed it himself. Good advice is good advice, and most people already know what good advice about their health will sound like - an iPod playing continuous loops of "eat better and exercise more" inside of a blowup doll is likely just as effective as any nerd in a white coat. Current Xander could take advice from even Barry because Xander needed to lose about seventy-five pounds more to become close to the super-sized Dr. Barry. That hit of the harsh truth in the form of advice can only acceptably come from a few sources, so reality is rarely given its needed opportunity, and the childish freedom to call someone fat to their face soon becomes lost behind social tact so obesity becomes easier to ignore. Even though most of my best friends are overweight, I would never toss them any unsolicited advice because being told to lose weight by even your best buddy will quickly turn that buddy into a distant acquaintance. I have just accepted the fact that our men's league basketball team is now mostly a squad of post-NBA TNT Charles Barkley's and the team is getting slower, jumping lower and becoming closer to being winless every year. There are only a few windows to get across the sentiment to care about personal health the right way, and if those windows are missed, the fight for fat self-awareness can be lost forever. Doctor visits are a window. Solicitation for advice is a window. This Taco Bell encounter was a window. I rolled into this restauarant just as the window opened.

"Alright, Dr. Grant, I will try to get active."

"Don't try, just do it. I hate working out just like anyone, but I do it anyway. Look at me, I'm a decrepit old man and I still work out almost every day."

"Come on, you're not that old."

"As old as your mother."

"Damn, that is old." Both Xander and I started laughing. Xander added, "Man, I wish you were still my doctor."

I slowed my laughter. That hypothetical chilled me. It is patients like Xander, people who were making themselves sick by one of the "too-much's" - eating too much, drinking too much or smoking too much - that made me choose pediatrics as my specialty in the first place. Pediatrics is about keeping kids healthy enough to live life; adult medicine is about slowing the progression to death. It's just hard to empathize with an adult that is the cause of their own morbid health. The too-much's are like skydiving. Is a skydiving death a tragedy? It may be sad for their loved ones, but it is not a tragedy. Skydiving's appeal is the adrenaline rush from tempting death, so when death answers now and then, it is not a shocking event. If some competent person is eating four thousand fried calories, drinking a couple cases of Keystone and smoking a carton of unfiltered every day, it is no tragedy when they heart attack out of this world.

"How is your mother doing, Xander?"

"She's doing well. I am actually just grabbing this quick dinner before I pick her up for our Friday movie night. We're going to see the latest Harold and Kumar. She loves those kinds of movies."

"That's hilarious."

"You should join us. Mom would love to see you."

"No, I can't. Thanks anyway, but I already have some plans tonight." I looked at my wristwatch for effect. "Ooh, for which I am extremely late. I better get going."

"Well, it was good seeing you, Dr. Grant."

"Good seeing you too, Xander. Say hi to your mom for me."

"Will do."

I turned towards the counter, as Xander dug into taco one of three. My mouth watered thinking about my order of three tacos and a burrito. Maybe even a Mexican pizza tonight. Now there's a fusion item. Where else can I get an Italian-Mexican entree? The smell of toasted processed corn shells and over-seasoned meat was comforting aromatherapy. I love Taco Bell.

DEAD

"I am so sorry, Kate."

With those words, she collapsed into my chest, sobbing
delicate mews. She smelled lightly of springtime. Her body
felt soft and warm like the insides of freshly baked French
bread. She was perfect in formfitting black from head to toe.
If you could ignore the casket in the front, all these bright
flowers and background classical music made this room feel like
a Sunday afternoon in the park with the Chicago Symphony
Orchestra.

I just kept rubbing her back in small circles. His death
was a real surprise. He was so young. Albert, that is.

He left a good looking corpse. Albert ran five miles every morning, was a Whole Foods health nut, and saw his doctor as recommended every year, always receiving a clean bill of health. I think the last time he ate a trans-fat was in high school. He gulped down a glass of red wine everyday after dinner in a single swallow like he was taking medicine just for its cardiac benefits, never considering savoring its more enjoyable qualities. A heart attack is not the way he should have gone - collapsing during an early morning run through the park. Though it does say a lot to what too much stress can do. This guy was a workaholic, a real type "A" personality, and loved chasing money. He could have retired comfortably with Kate years ago, but he loved the drive of making a buck. A hundred hour work week was just a normal week by Al. Take that grind times thirty some years and you've got the makings of a Heart Attack Jones.

"Hi, Dr. Grant."

I looked to my left and it was Xander, coming towards me in a Rascal. He looked like a garbage bag overfilled with dirt being pushed down the street in a motorized wheelbarrow. His banding looked like it was failing terribly. He was much bigger. And had a poorly kempt beard. With cookie crumbs stuck in it. He must eat like Cookie Monster, with more crumbs spewing out than being swallowed. There was an *US Weekly* and a

OK! magazine in the rascal's front basket. It looks like this
guy was now consuming processed trash down both the gullet and
into the noodle, regardless of occasion. His motorized approach
did end Kate's hug, and she started wiping away her tears and
trying for some composure.

"Hi Xander."

"Thanks for coming, Dr. Grant, it is good to see you."

"I am so sorry about your dad. He was a good guy."

"Thanks, Dr. Grant, I really appreciate it."

Silence. Kate sniffed. I heard Xander's stomach growling.

"So, what is the deal with the Rascal, are you hurt or
something?"

Xander let out a soft laugh. "Even here you're worried
about me. You are one of a kind, Dr. Grant, one of a kind."

"I thought you'd be running marathons by now."

"I thought so too, but a few weeks ago, I thought I was
ready to run a mile, but after a few hundred yards, my knees
said no way. It hurts to just walk now."

He lifted up his right pant leg and showed off an elastic
knee brace. Fat and skin squeezed through the circular kneecap
opening at the center of the brace, looking like a just-about-
to-pop pimple. His leg skin looked like he had been wearing a
tourniquet for days -- a purple mess of venous insufficiency.

He continued, "And then my dad died, so I pretty much spent a week in front of the TV with frozen pizzas on a sheet pan, a pizza cutter in my left hand, and my right hand going sheet pan to mouth."

Kate added, in a tattling tone, "And he ate about a million Reeses Pieces."

"No mom, it was regular M&M's in a jar of peanut butter and a spoon. Get it right." Then Xander laughed. The suspension on his Rascal creaked with his heaving guffaws. "I was actually doing great for a while. I got under three hundred pounds for the first time since high school. Don't worry, I'll get back. Just like the people in these magazines."

Unlikely. Xander was now in the classification of a failed surgical intervention. This guy was put under anesthesia, incised, had a camera and some rods poked into his abdomen, then had a silicone strip placed around the top portion of his stomach to create a change purse for food, and he still couldn't keep off the weight. And now He was on a Rascal, using external energy and engineering to do the equivalent of walking. Of course it was shocking that Albert had beat Xander to death. Though, with the way he's going, it doesn't seem like it will be by that much. My bet is that tomorrow, Xander's going to be cruising on his Rascal, sloppily eating an Italian beef with

sweet peppers, then suddenly slump down into its soft leather
seat, his Italian beef falling to the sidewalk, dead of a heart
attack as the Rascal slowly rolls into the front door of a
Krispy Kreme.

"I am sure you will get back, Xander."

Kate was still tearing a bit, so I gave her a half hug with
my left arm over her right shoulder, which she leaned into a
resting of her right temple against my shoulder and staring off
into nowhere.

Xander looked over at his dad's casket. "Being fit sure
didn't help him."

I looked down at Kate on my shoulder. She was spaced and
didn't hear Xander. The comment made some backward sense. If a
healthy guy like Al can die of a heart attack so young, why even
try to get healthy? Why should someone deprive themselves the
joys of butter and sugar when eating nothing but twigs and
berries still might not matter for longevity? Because even
though fit people can die early and obese people can live a long
time, being healthy is about reducing risk, not eliminating it.
No one can eliminate all risk. Albert still had his stress. If
I were pulling playing Russian roulette, I would want the
minimum number of bullets in the chambers as I could negotiate.
If one is the minimum, then one is what I would want. Zero

would of course be better, but then it wouldn't be Russian
roulette. Eliminating all risk would make life not a life. I
can sit inside a sealed bubble getting tube fed a slurry of
calories, vitamins and minerals and live to a hundred and fifty,
but then, why am I even here? You have to eat some bacon, or
dig into a good chunk of chocolate cake, or eat way too much at
a buffet once in a while. Food is meant to be enjoyed. But,
swimming every day in a sea of bacon cheeseburgers and chili
fries and chocolate milkshakes doesn't make much sense either.
Who wants to play Russian roulette with six in the chamber?
That's just suicide. Xander has had six in the chamber for a
while now and all that was left was for death to pull the
trigger.

Xander nodded and then rolled his Rascal towards Albert's
casket. I steered Kate towards a chair and sat next to her as
she started crying again. She was using my dress shirt as her
personal tissue. Bad idea to go with my best white dress shirt
today. Just as Xander reached the head of the casket, he looked
back at us and smirked - his mom's head was burying deeper into
his old pediatrician's chest at his dad's wake. Xander just
stared at Albert for a while, until some random family member
interrupted his condolence to offer their own condolences.

Xander was looking at the tip of his downward spiral in Albert's pale corpse. Accelerating life turned rotting meat. Albert went much too soon, Xander was living on borrowed time, but he was treating his rental like he didn't care because he didn't own it, playing whiffle ball with his RedBox DVD. He was still young enough to change, but he was also old enough to have started setting his behaviors into a lifestyle. The opportunity for change was slipping quickly as hardening concrete.

The condolences to Xander from passing friends and family were initially made in quiet earnest, but there was a moment in each exchange when their words became parsed in escalating awkwardness at the realization that Xander reeked of death. He was tinged gray, diaphoretic, in mild respiratory distress and emanated fungal gas. Standard wake prepositional rhetoric of "at peace" or "in a happier place now" was just as applicable to mean death would be the only relief to a young man left to motor on a scooter from gross mass grown during a life of over-consumption.

Kate's body heaved deeper into my chest. She felt fragile, as if a whiff of breeze would send her to the ground. I gave the top of her head a little peck.

Then the carpet matting trembled with a bang. Albert was still resting quietly in the casket. The Rascal was empty and

decelerating driverless down the center aisle. A rush of dark
dress formed a large semicircle around the heap of flesh.

"Is he having a heart attack?"

"He's still breathing, I think."

"Get him some water!"

"His blood sugar might be low, grab some cookies!"

"Is there a doctor here?"

Kate's head lifted and she gave my thigh a squeeze, nodding
in Xander's direction. I ambled over with Kate. By that time,
Xander was already sitting up and trying to get up.

"Hey, buddy, are you all right?"

"Yeah, Dr. Grant, I'm okay." He stood up with a grunt.

"What happened?"

"I tried standing up to give my uncle a hug and I felt
dizzy and hot then blacked out. Maybe my blood sugar is low?"

Someone instantly handed him a cookie and he chewed it
down. It sounded like a simple vasovagal episode, just his
heart rate and/or blood pressure dropping temporarily from
triggered brainstem activation and nothing to do with blood
sugar, but I didn't feel the need to give some lengthy
exposition to these strangers on his correct diagnosis and why
the blood sugar theory was incorrect, especially since he was
recovered now. I just shrugged at his question.

"I better get something to eat before this happens again."

One of the onlookers brought the Rascal back to Xander. He huffed his was back onto the seat and motored out the front door towards the buffet.

Kate mouthed "thank you" and gave me a peck on the cheek.

GOLF

I play golf. A lot. As much as I hate the stereotype of
the doctor distractedly rushing through patients to get to the
golf course, I got bit by the golf bug early in my childhood and
just kept on playing. I'm a golfer that became a doctor, not
the other way around. I love the immediate consequence for any
given action, the never-ending battle with the defeatist mind,
and the perpetual search for elusive perfection amidst a sea of
failure. Makes me wonder why I went into a profession where I
deal with patients who don't care about consequences of stroking
out at age fifty as long as they can eat their hamburger and
fries today, parents that believe they need no more information
to engage their minds because they equate surfing a few random
blogs for a few hours on par with a lifetime of medical

training, and patients that expect perfect health in perpetuity regardless of the fact they just spent their failing health sucking Marlboros and Bud Light in between bites of deep fried anything while lying on the couch day to night. Now that I am retired, what else is there to do but forget about medicine and play the greatest game every day?

So I am here at the club this morning, like I am almost every morning, ready to get in a quick 18. Today, I'm waiting for Xander. Ever since he got well enough to get out of his Rascal, Kate has been begging me to take Xander out to the course, to get him active and exercising in something, even if it is the slow burn of golf. I usually like walking my round, sometimes with a caddie if I'm feeling tired, just to maximize the physical aspects of the game. No caddie for me today, though. Xander rolled up to the first tee today in a cart. He was already sweated through his XXXL polo, his wrinkled ballooning shorts cinched on with an belt that bulged oddly at the buckle form the extra holes punched into it, and he looked badly out of breath.

"Hey, Dr. Grant, ready to crush some rocks?"

"Sounds good. Are you going to walk or take that cart?"

"Cart, for sure. Do you want to get in?"

"No thanks, Xander, I am just going to walk it."

This was working out okay. With him in the cart and me walking, I could at least get some sporadic separation and concentrate on my own game, instead of him being in my ear all day, a foot away from me. Ninety percent of golf is getting to your next shot, so if we shared that cart, even in a quick four hour round, it could've meant over three and a half hours of face-to-face time with Xander. Not the way I want to play my golf. Plus, maybe with the cart I wouldn't have to resuscitate him on the third green.

The first hole is a short par four that doglegs a little to the left, and the tee shot landing area is guarded by a couple of bunkers on either side of the fairway. Most people lay up short of the trouble, about a 240 pop to a wider fairway, but I like trying to cut the corner with a driver, and this hole fits my standard draw, so I always take a good rip. I only successfully cut the corner about thirty percent of the time, of which today was thankfully one of those three in ten.

Xander stepped up to the box with his driver too. He used to be a good golfer back on his high school team, when he was in the midst of his slimmer phase, and even got to the state finals one year. He now took a cut at the ball looking like he had never played before. His swing was now a series of compensations to get around his massive chest and belly. His

setup was further away from the ball than should be, and he had
hunch of a bend in his posture, to accommodate the extra mass
resting on thighs and hanging between arm and ball. The
takeaway was round and flat and stopped short, with a slow
weight shift, then quickly to a big over-the-top move, getting
the club in front of his belly with a glacial lateral shift of
weight back towards his left foot, with just a hint of a proper
forward turn. He did use the ground for leverage well and did a
proper post-up to his left leg, but his swing was a supreme
digger, always leaving two divots: a rectangular one from his
club into ground, and a circular one under his left shoe from
twisting all of his weight onto his left foot, as if an elephant
stamping out a cigarette butt. Xander's hand-eye coordination
was impressive that he could even make contact with the ball
with all of his moving parts. Even if he caught it flush, I
doubt it would've made it to the bunkers. He duck-hooked this
drive low and left, just into the rough short of the left
fairway bunker.

He waddled back into the cart, reached into a cooler for a
beer and stuck a stogie into his mouth. It was just past nine
o'clock. This is not a good step towards real exercise. Four
hours lugging a thirty pound bag over five miles of rolling
hills while stopping every so often to swing metal into rubber

is good exercise. Letting a motorized vehicle lug person and clubs over five miles of rolling asphalt while stopping every so often to suck back beers and cigars between swings of metal into rubber is barely exercise at all. Xander is using golf as exercise in word only – he was going to probably gain weight during today's round.

I chunked a little wedge to the front fringe of the green. Xander proceeded to hit three more low skanks, and twenty minutes later finally skulled his ball onto the green. It had taken us as a twosome thirty minutes to get to the green. At this rate we would finish our eighteen in over nine hours. I looked around and thanked the golf gods that the course was empty of other players.

Two putts later I was in for par. Xander lined up his putt standing, addressed his ball with elbows resting on his love handles, took a whack with all wrist, and banged it home off the back lip of the cup.

"Yeah, baby!"

As he gleefully shuffled the twenty-five feet to pick his ball from the cup, he left deep foot indentations with each step on the dew-softened greens. I hope every group that plays on this green after us today doesn't mind putting over size twelve craters. The deepest footprint was left right by the hole as

Xander leaned all of his weight onto his left foot when he bent

over to pick his Titleist from the cup, nearly falling flat on

his face, but catching himself at the last moment by gouging the

butt end his putter into the green, leaving yet another pock

mark. As he walked back to his cart, more imprints in the dew

trailed just behind him, and he was casually using his putter as

a cane, so now half the green had tripod stamps of feet and the

bottom of a putter.

The second hole is a short par three with a marsh fronting

the green and a large bunker hugging the back. There is a bit

of elevation to get to the tee box, which is a pain to walk

because the stone stairs were built steeply, but Xander just

pressed his pedal down flat and got his cart to lurch up the

incline without effort. He finished his first beer and popped

into another just as I put my bag down behind the right tee

marker. I teed off first and skulled one into the back bunker.

Xander chuckled, "Beach!" as he bent over to tee his ball.

Xander suddenly jerked, grabbed his back and instantly crumpled

to the ground. He was writhing in pain. I glanced at my ball

in the back bunker in case the falling Xander ground shake from

a hundred and twenty yards away popped the ball backwards onto

the green. It hadn't. I looked back at Xander and his writhing was rubbing the grass bald on the tee box. Golf was over for Xander today after one hole.

As he gingerly got back up, Xander grunted, "Dr. Grant, could you get me my pills from the cart?"

There was a prescription bottle in one of the cup holders. Vicodin. I walked the bottle back over to Xander and he popped his last two pills and swallowed with just saliva.

"When did you start taking Vicodin, Xander?"

"Last year sometime. My joints have been killing me for a while. Don't really know why. Glad I had some left for my back today."

I caught myself laughing. He should be in pain. He's always going to have pain. No human body would ever be able to be abused that much and remain unscathed. The Vicodin is trying to do its part to ease the pain, while Xander does nothing himself to lessen the cause of the pain, even by a pound. He's probably in actuality increasing the pain by pounds every week. I'm betting he has had to up the pain medicine potency exponentially with his weight. He probably started with some over-the-counter stuff, then to some lower potency prescription meds, and then as the dosing started getting maxed-out and tolerance started to build, he went on the prescription medicine up-shuffle for more potency. I hoped his delusion as to the cause of his pain wasn't making him too dependent on narcotics, and he was now using doctors as a drug seeker. Drug-seekers: the scum of the Earth. These are people that try to use the helpful nature of medical professionals as a vulnerability and hop from different doctors to clinics to emergency rooms and make up any story to get their fix of prescribable narcotics. Uh, I have an uncontrollable migraine that somehow no medication made specifically for migraines can lessen and I don't want to take anything or do anything to prevent these migraines so I need only the most potent narcotics to alleviate this pain that I rate ten out of ten as I am explaining my condition without any apparent distress. Or, uh, I am a 300 lbs. slug with sketchy work accident related back pain that didn't prevent me from casually ambling to this clinic, but has now worsened to such a degree precisely at the entrance of this clinic that I cannot move and can only cry out in pain. Or, uh, I somehow lost my prescription bottle full of narcotic or it was stolen during a recent home robbery, and now I need some emergency meds for my fibromyalgia until I can see my regular doctor, and even though when you checked the state prescription monitoring database with my exact name and birth date it showed that I have filled multiple prescriptions for this narcotic in the last few weeks from multiple doctors from different clinics across the

region, I don't know what those prescriptions are and it could
be a case of identity theft where the thief used my name to fill
the exact narcotic I am currently asking for now. The whine
that these people are suffering from some addiction disease that
makes their lies beyond their control is absurd, as if their
deceit was part of their DNA and some basic human drive akin to
breathing. The real disease is sociopathy - persons unable to
consider anything other than getting what they want. They are
consciously deciding drug addicts, actively directing all their
human resources to scheme for their next high at the expense of
all others. Series of poor decisions become behavior and
habit, then lifestyle. Similarly, some claim the obese to be
drug seekers of the drug of food, the excuse being that this is
an addiction where one is forced to take some of the drug
everyday just to live and that a ham sandwich is in the same
vein as crack cocaine. If obesity really was a disease
comprised of some uncontrollable urge to eat, then the obese
would be real world zombies, mindlessly trolling for their food
with empty abandon and all human free thought removed, not
caring that they are inflicting increasing pain with every
mouthful. Forty to fifty percent of the US population is obese,
so if this zombie epidemic were the case, this country would be
living a dystopia filled with drooling, disfigured humanoids

with no other drive than to devour hamburgers and fries. But, everyone has a choice what they put into their mouths. No one is force fed fat. As it is, the obese are simple over-consumers in a society of over-consumption with poorly developed eating habits and poorly developed self-control, continuing their lifestyle by justifying every calorie bomb in their minds as entitled sustenance and excusing their appearance with nonsense: uh, I have a slow metabolism or, uh, I'm big boned or, uh, I'm too busy to exercise. The active, ongoing choice to repeatedly over-consume consequence in early death, humiliation, and negative social stigmas. The world could use less consuming.

   As Xander stood leaning against his cart, he started rambling, "You know, Dr. Grant, I had a weird dream last night. I was at a party at Arnold Palmer's house, and was stuffing myself with all the hors d'oeuvres I could find. I then took a tray of pigs in a blanket and snuck away into one of his bedrooms. A little kid was napping in the bed, so I jostled the kid awake and literally kicked him out of the room. I snuggled myself into the sheets and started popping the pigs into my mouth, and they were so greasy that I had to wipe my hands on the white sheets. I must've eaten at least a few dozen. After I finished, I fell asleep and rolled off the bed onto the floor. As I snapped awake, Arnold Palmer burst into the door and asked where his grandson went. I said I didn't know. Then he asked who had made the mess on the bed. I looked and the bed's sheets were yellow and brown with grease. I said it was probably his grandson's mess. Arnold gave my greasy face a look of disdain and just left. That was my dream. Maybe it means I should give up golf."

Xander's subconscious was a mess of shame. The dream of Xander bullying a child and befouling the golfing King's bedroom sheets because of food should have at least warranted consideration that the dream was about food and his ills, but instead he interpreted it as a signal to give up golf, as if Arnold Palmer's reaction to having the culprit of his greased sheets try to cover up his disgusting actions with an obvious lie was just about Arnie, as an embodiment of golf, frowning at Xander. Maybe all Senator Larry Craig's troubles were just a sign for him to limit expelling his waste to his bathroom at home rather than public restrooms. I just shrugged back a smirk at Xander.

As he gingerly got into his golf cart, he uttered between grunts, "Dr. Grant, my back is pretty messed up, I'm just going to head for the clubhouse. I have to get a refill for more pain pills to pop or I'm going to be bedridden. Sorry, I couldn't finish with you."

I shrugged again, but with a smile. No need to apologize for that. This day just got a lot lighter.

Xander popped another beer as he reversed back down the hill, then turned the cart back towards the clubhouse. As he disappeared down the cart path, I teed up another ball, for practice. I popped it up into the marsh. Whatever. I grabbed the plastic seed dispenser from next to the tee marker, poured turf seed over the missing grass from my divot and where Xander had writhed bald, then picked up my bag and headed towards the green.

Another great day for golf. Maybe I'll play 54 today.

WEDDING

Xander was supposed to scooter his mom down the aisle for our wedding. A destination wedding in Maui makes for a selfishly inconvenient and small wedding, so Xander was a big part of the ceremony's plans, all 420 lbs. of him. But, this was the weekend he decided to be patchy with his insulin administration and go on a luau bender. It was real suspicious when he didn't show up for the rehearsal dinner, when the last dinner he missed might have been so I wasn't too shocked when Kate's sister found him passed out in his hotel room, breath smelling like a fruit basket. So we postponed the wedding a week while Xander got tuned up at the hospital.

When we went to visit him the day before he was first scheduled to be discharged, he was just starting his lunch. I saw a salad on his bed tray. It looked great for hospital food:

crisp spring greens, bright cherry tomatoes, dewy cucumbers, julienned carrots, baby peas, cubed beets, and a wedge of pineapple on the side. Then Xander proceeded to rip open two large dressing packets and drench the greens with ranch – it was now ranch soup with a sprinkling of salad. When the farmer put all that care into the months of planting, growing and harvesting the perfect vegetable, little did he know that it would be used as a garnish for processed fat.

The scene reminds me of a grocery trip I made about five years ago, when I last saw Xander attempting to be healthy in the flesh. He was strolling through Whole Foods with a cart full of oranges, grapefruit and strawberries, stopping by the grain dispensers and filling up a green plastic tube bag with organic oats. A three hundred and fifty pound guy at Whole Foods pushing around a cart filled with the groceries of a one hundred pound vegan woman. I continued to follow him to see what else he tossed into his cart. I don't know what was more ridiculous: an old man peering around stacks of organic navel oranges and cheeses at a fat man's grocery shopping or Xander at Whole Foods. He slowly meandered through more departments, like a barge rolling down the Chicago River, and continued by tossing a couple ready-made Indian frozen meals into the cart, passing by the pastries and cakes, eating a sample of some sharp white

cheddar, grabbing a loaf of whole wheat artesian bread, downing
a sample of some whole grain crackers, getting a pound of sliced
deli turkey meat, and then he started heading for the checkout.
As he loaded his items onto the conveyor belt, while I watched
from behind a stack of natural dye free bar soap, I thought of
how he must go home, cut his fruit into slices, arrange them
between two slices of whole wheat bread alongside some turkey,
dip the sandwich in butter and coat them in oats, then deep-fry
the whole mess in chocolate sauce, and eventually down it
drenched in ranch dressing. There is no way three hundred and
fifty pounds are maintained with what he had in his shopping
cart. This hospital salad is how big numbers can be maintained
with healthy foods.

I blurted, "Xander, take it easy on the dressing, you're
ruining the salad."

"Alright, alright, I will, but salad tastes like crap
without this much ranch." Xander smirked, then continued, "Hey
wait a minute, you're not my dad yet, so I don't have to listen
to that." Xander started laughing as he threw a forkful down
the hatch.

Later that night, while Kate and I were having dinner, the
physician taking care of him, Dr. Reebs, called and said
Xander's sugars had gotten too high again. They had noticed him

looking more tired that afternoon and when they checked his blood sugar, it was 650. A nurse found some empty candy wrappers stuffed underneath his mattress - two king size Snickers, a Kit Kat, Milky Way and Twix. His discharge would have to be postponed. So we postponed our wedding another few days.

Postponing for more time in paradise is a terrific consolation. Xander's laissez-faire attitude about his diabetes is just giving Kate and I opportunity to stay in Maui longer. Our guest list was shrinking with every delay, but no matter to us. Xander was the reason we got to Maui in the first place.

After Albert died, Kate got despondent. Xander told me that she didn't leave her bedroom for a month. But somehow, he got her to leave the house by enticing her with golf, a game their whole family used to play together when he was a kid. Xander's golf days were long over, as he hasn't been able to coil a golf club around his body since cracking four hundred pounds soon after our couple holes together at the club, but he started riding in a cart while Kate walked eighteen. Kate's mood started to lighten while walking fairways and greens. And Xander started inviting me to join their twosome. Eighteen holes once a week meant spending a few hours together once a week. That soon became playing eighteen a few times a week,

which became post-round dinners a few times a week, became
dinner and a movie on weekends, and became spending nights in
with just me and Kate. That first night I spent overnight with
Kate, Xander was there the next morning in the kitchen, dropping
off a vase of fresh flowers for Kate's dining room table, like
he did every day since Albert died, and just quipped to me with
a grin, "Hey, step-dad." And he was right; I asked Kate if I
could become Xander's step-dad a couple months later.

The Maui wedding was all Xander too. He was going to pay
for our wedding and make it a five star affair. Kate and I
fought him on it - we were both well enough along to pay for it
ourselves - but Xander insisted, and said it would be his
wedding present to us. So here we were in a Honeymoon Suite at
the Four Seasons and Xander was putzing around in a 12x8
hospital room. He didn't seem to be doing much to change that
situation, though.

The nurse started noticing Xander was getting overly winded
when he got up to go to the bathroom. Initially, no one thought
anything of it - someone weighing four-fifty was not going to
impress with physical endurance. But, it started to get worse,
where he started looking sweaty and pale, as if he just ran a
marathon, after going to urinate. The doctor eventually ordered
an echocardiogram. His heart was less squeezing than just

jiggling in his chest. Xander had heart failure. He was
struggling to pump out enough oxygen-rich blood to meet the
demands of his mass and vital organs. What he needed was an
elephant heart pumping in his chest.

His health had been going downhill for the past few years
before this latest finding, especially in the last few months,
but he hated going to the doctor and he hated taking medicine,
so he just toughed out his fatigue and general malaise
regardless of anyone's urging to go take care of himself better.
That sentiment had been echoed by too many for so long that it
was white noise to him. He was a grown man, after all, able to
decide for himself whether to take his insulin and Metformin
everyday instead of spending every waking minute on the couch
watching every season of *Lost* back-to-back whilst downing two
entire XXL cheese pizzas in one sitting. Now this grown man is
stuck sickly on this island.

Xander fast deteriorated. His sugars got harder to control
and the doctors were having a hard time finding the right
cocktail of medications to get his heart pumping better. Then
he had a heart attack - a full coronary artery blowout at age
forty-two. He got intubated, which took the head of anesthesia
ten attempts due to Xander's obstructive neck fat. Machines
took over the basic human functions that define life and turned

him into a mass whose only ability was to produce urine and stool. He even had to get fed through a central line, getting his vitamins and calories from a yellowish slurry one drip at a time. This was how he was going to go, without even his greatest love.

The level of love Xander had for food was awesome. He passed on women, happiness and health - passed on life - to be with food. Food was the mistress that enticed him to lie and justify and cheat to the point of self-loathing. Food was the selfish mistress that only wanted Xander to herself, so she slowly fashioned him a fat man suit so he would never get other real opportunities to find or attract other loves. Xander stayed with food as his lover even though he knew that with his level of infatuation, food would also be his executioner. Would I be with Kate if I knew that the more I loved her, the more likely it is that she would smother me in my sleep? Food was crazier. Food was never sated with Xander's love, and stalked him at every turn, constantly sending him pangs of messages that he always needed to have more. Xander will eventually have loved food to death. I have never loved anything as much as Xander has loved food. Not many have.

Not even close.

www.ingramcontent.com/pod-product-compliance
Lightning Source LLC
Chambersburg PA
CBHW070853120626
46556CB00002B/968